WomanStyle

Dressing Rich

Traveling Light

*Dress Like a Million
(on Considerably Less)*

DOES THIS MAKE ME LOOK FAT?

DOES THIS MAKE ME LOOK FAT?

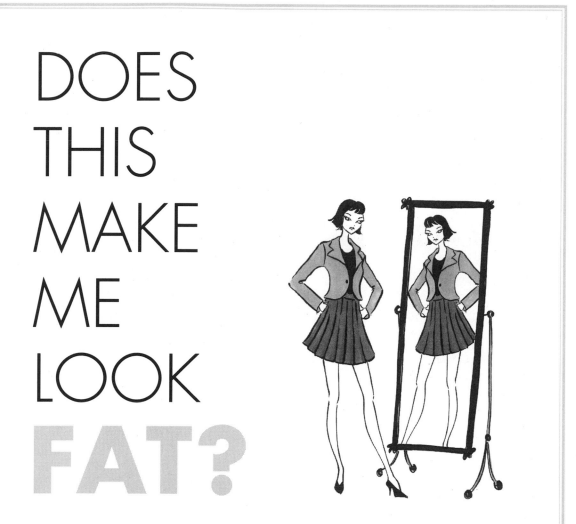

THE DEFINITIVE RULES FOR DRESSING THIN FOR EVERY HEIGHT, SIZE, AND SHAPE

LEAH FELDON

ILLUSTRATIONS BY LEIGH ANN DAVIS

VILLARD ❧ NEW YORK

All rights reserved under International and Pan-American Copyright Conventions.
Published in the United States by Villard Books, a division of Random House, Inc.,
New York, and simultaneously in Canada by Random House of Canada Limited,
Toronto.

VILLARD BOOKS and colophon are registered trademarks of Random House, Inc.

Grateful acknowledgment is made to Dwarf Music for permission to reprint
six lines from "Leopard-Skin Pill-Box Hat" by Bob Dylan. Copyright © 1966
by Dwarf Music. Reprinted by permission.

Library of Congress Cataloging-in-Publication Data

Feldon, Leah
Does this make me look fat?: the definitive rules for dressing thin/Leah Feldon.
p.   cm.
ISBN 0-375-50361-7 (alk. paper)
1. Clothing and dress.   2. Fashion.   3. Overweight persons—Costume.
I. Title: Definitive rules for dressing thin.   II. Title.

TT507.F432   2000
646'.3—dc21   99-49565

Villard website address: www.villard.com
Printed in the United States of America on acid-free paper
9 8 7 6 5 4 3 2
First Edition
BOOK DESIGN BY JO ANNE METSCH

To my family, and to all women—large, small, and in between—everywhere

ACKNOWLEDGMENTS

My sincere thanks to all those who so generously contributed their energies: Stedman Mays, my fabulous agent, for his brilliance, style, and unfailing good humor; Leigh Ann Davis, my new best friend, for her wonderful illustrations and for being such a doll to work with; my husband, Adam Mitchell, also for being a doll, and for his dedicated proofreading and all those extra commas; my enlightened editor, Mollie Doyle, for totally getting it on every level; Dan Rembert, Melody Guy, Martha Schwartz, and the rest of the superb team at Villard for their great work; Jason Baruch for his astute legal advice; Rachel Kahan for her knowledgeable support; my sisters, Eda Baruch and Debbie Kahan, and Rob Kinch Manuel, Jean-Charles Duchene, Nancy Ganz, Lis Loeb, and Diane Cambareri, for sharing their respective expertise; and my mother, Henrietta Kahan, for her lifelong dedication to my cause . . . still stylish after all these years.

CONTENTS

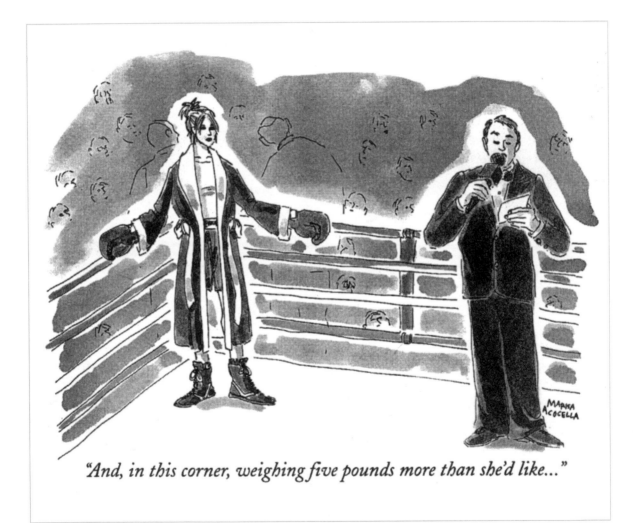

"And, in this corner, weighing five pounds more than she'd like..."

DOES THIS MAKE ME LOOK FAT?

I cannot tell a lie. Sometimes even I feel fat and bloated.

—NAOMI CAMPBELL, supermodel

INTRODUCTION

> *I don't think the rules ever change. People want to look taller and thinner. No one says, "Ooh! Let me buy that dress because it makes me feel matronly!"*
>
> —MICHAEL KORS, designer

One day not too long ago, while I was in the dressing room of one of my favorite stores, trying to figure out just which, of the all the black pants I had in there, was *the* perfect pair, I heard the woman next door chatting with her saleslady. Since I was rather preoccupied, their conversation was just background buzz until I heard the woman ask loud and clear, "Does this make me look fat?" Hey, I thought, *that's just what I was thinking!*

Now, truly, I'm not what you'd call fat. Neither was the other woman. I sneaked a peek at her when I left, and she looked like a blond Julia Roberts. But you know what? When it comes to self-perception, size doesn't matter. **We all feel fat, or think we look fat, at one time or another, no matter what size we are!** I must have heard the phrase "Does this make look fat?" a gazillion times during my twenty-odd years in the fashion business—from every size woman imaginable.

If you've picked up this book, you've probably said, "Does this make me look fat?" too. And you might not even be close to fat! You could be one of those women who people think are totally nuts

when they even mention the F-word. Or you could be average. Or you could be a plus size. It really doesn't matter—being fat or feeling fat, in a crazy way, it's all the same. We stare in the mirror and focus on every little bump, bulge, and protuberance until our body looks like a Himalayan landscape to us. We all know this is not particularly healthy, but we do it anyway.

There's no sense in me trying to talk you out of your neurosis, as I've been trying to talk myself out of mine for years. It's a fruitless endeavor. (I'm fairly sure a twenty-five-year ascetic meditation retreat would set me straight, but who has the time?) So what to do? We switch to plan B and handle the problem in the time-honored American tradition—we cover up whatever's making us crazy. We disguise it. We make it go away. You can't be too neurotic about something that you can't see.

All we have to do is choose the right clothes—clothes that camouflage any real or imagined figure flaws rather than highlighting them—and learn how to do it with style. **That's what I call *Camouflage Chic!***

When you think about it, there are really only two kinds of clothes in the world—those that make you look fat and those that don't. All the rest is just details. There are, of course, degrees within those two categories. In the *fat-maker* category, there are some clothes that will make you just a teensy-weensy bit heftier and others that will pack on an extra five pounds. And in the *nonfat* category, there are clothes that are virtually neutral and those that can make you look five pounds skinnier. This book is about zeroing in on the last kind. *Does This Make Me Look Fat?* is dedicated to the proposition that we'd all rather wear clothes that render us slimmer as opposed to heavier—and while we're at it, taller rather than shorter. Fact is, tall and slim is a good look.

Before I go any further, let me nip any potential dissension in the bud and slip in a disclaimer for any plus-size lobbyers out there who may be tempted to pick on me for not taking a total "Big Is Beautiful" stance here, as well as for any hard-line feminists who feel this entire subject is demeaning and that we women should be judged not by how we look but rather by our brains, character, and mettle.

To the first group let me say that big may be beautiful, but it can be even more lovely with effective camouflaging. Nobody—be they size sixteen or size six—wants to look heavier than they actually are. That's just a given. I've dressed a lot of women over the years and not one has ever asked me to help them look shorter or stockier. And yes, we should absolutely learn to love and accept ourselves as we are—warts, potbellies, and all. But who says we have to exhibit those features to the world at large?

And to my feminist sisters, let me say that I agree with you wholeheartedly. We should not be judged by our appearance . . . but we are, so get over it. It's been that way since cave babes started wearing fur. This book is egalitarian—it's for all women of all sizes (and of all political persuasions) who want their clothes to work for them instead of against them. It's as simple as that.

> In the end, fashion is not such a silly thing. Even if you say you don't dress, it's not true. Either way, you make a choice.
>
> —MIUCCIA PRADA, designer

Here *fat* is a relative term, used in the purely unclinical, semiobsessive, sartorially savvy, fun-loving sense of the word. It doesn't matter whether you're five ounces over your fighting weight, thirty pounds overweight, or just want to make that totally fit body of yours look as sleek as possible. If you really want the answer to "Does this make me look fat?" this is where you'll get it—no holds barred. Here, clothes that add heft are taken to task and those that diminish it are cheered. In these pages you will find out exactly what you need to know to make you look slimmer, taller, and better proportioned in your clothes. (Out of clothes, I'm afraid you're on your own.)

A truth-in-advertising moment: The information in this book is not going to transform a 160-pound woman into Kate Moss or a five-foot, one-inch woman into Xena, Warrior Princess. This is, after all, a fashion book, not a "Course in Miracles." But it can help you knock off a few *virtual* pounds, grow an extra *virtual* vertical inch or two, look generally sleeker, and make your fashion life a lot easier.

When it comes to camouflaging, most of us have heard about the perils of wearing broad horizontal stripes (eek!) and the like, but that's just the tip of the iceberg. There are a slew of other camouflaging principles that are much more subtle—and just as important. In my workshops, participants are constantly amazed at the difference a simple placement of buttons, the shape of a lapel, the width of a strap, or a slight shift in color tone can make on the girth meter. It's not a religious experience exactly, but it definitely changes the way these women see clothes and the way they buy them. Best of all, it's knowledge they can use for the rest of their lives, because the principles are timeless and apply to whatever new cards fashion may deal us.

> *I started very early to believe in an inside-out concept—that if you look as good as you can, you will feel better.*
>
> —JIL SANDER, designer

There's another dimension here too: There's a real feeling of empowerment that comes from knowing what's right for you and wearing clothes that perfectly suit your body. You simply feel better about yourself. I'll offer myself up here as case in point: I have two pairs of slim black pants, one that fits me perfectly and makes me look trim and slender, and the other that's a bit snug and makes my stomach look paunchy. Even though I wear the snug ones only with a roomy top that covers the offending paunch, I know it's lurking under there, and I *feel* fat when I wear the pants. I don't feel as self-assured as I do in my slim pants. **How you feel in clothes is as important as how you look in them.** When you *feel* confident, you *look* confident.

> *All we can do is maintain—we can't fight aging. . . . Women have to accept that our bodies give in to gravity. That's life.*
>
> —EVE LOM, skin-care entrepreneur

I've been using the concept of fashion camouflage for more than twenty years: first as a stylist, designer, and image consultant, then as a journalist, author, and television commentator and host. I've dealt with fashion from every angle—behind the camera, in front of the camera, in production meetings, and on the computer screen. I've dressed models, celebrities, and real people. And if there's one thing I've learned in all these years, it's this: **While clothes don't make the woman, they sure do help.** *Any figure can be improved with the right clothes.* And the *right* clothes don't necessarily cost more than *wrong* ones. You can buy totally nonfat clothes for the same amount of money you spend on clothes that are the equivalent of a double chocolate shake. It's all in your choices.

A lot of what makes a choice the right one is *proportion*. The first time I saw Matthew McConaughey on the big screen, for instance, I wasn't thinking, Oh, isn't he darling! like all the other women in the audience. I was thinking, My god, he is sooo long-waisted! And Sharon Stone—I can't watch her without thinking, Great proportions! I'm a proportion nut. Balance is one of the first things I see when I look at someone. I notice if their necklines are shortening their necks or their hemlines are lengthening their legs, and everything else in between.

Actually, my mother says I've always been this way. She remembers us all sitting poolside in Florida, when I was about eight, and me emphatically declaring that my pudgy five-year-old brother would look "really tons better" in boxer trunks than in his little Speedo—which, of course, was true. (My brother's pudginess, for the record, is long gone . . . and he now wears boxers.)

Anyway, my keen eye—or dubious talent, however you choose to look at it—has come in quite handy over the years. I'm hoping now it can be a big help to you. Although we'll be focusing on looks that slim and trim here, we'll always be touching on the timeless tenets of good taste and style as well, which is the *chic* part of Camouflage Chic. As you read, think about the kind of things you like to wear, what you feel most comfortable in, and the kind of lifestyle you lead. Then apply the rules and adapt some of the style ideas here to shape—or re-shape—your wardrobe and personal style.

> *I've known women who wouldn't be considered conventionally beautiful but because of their self-confidence and humor, they're the hottest women in the room. Conversely, I've known gorgeous women whose mouths you just want to cover with duct tape.*
>
> —KIRSTEN JOHNSTON, actress

My goals here are threefold: 1. The next time you ask, "Does this make me look fat?" you will be able to correctly answer the question *instantly;* 2. you will not waste money on things you'll never wear or waste time trying on everything in your closet every time you get dressed in the eternal search for the least fattening outfit; and 3. you will have enough information under your belt to "just say no" to any tempting new trends that may look fetching on a fourteen-year-old, but will make you look awful.

One last word before we get going: I'm generally not big on rules—especially traditional fashion rules. You'll never hear me telling anyone they can wear patent leather only after Memorial Day, or no white before Memorial Day, or absolutely no velvet until 5:00 P.M. Who made those up, anyway? It's a mystery. The good news is that whoever did probably isn't around anymore, so who cares? **The only**

fashion rules that count, as far as I'm concerned, are those based on common sense and those that we can use to *our* advantage—and for our specific purposes here, that means rules that can help give us the shape we want: the Rules of Camouflage Chic. These rules are time-tested and universal tenets that can give you the flattering look of the "right" proportions. All the great couturiers know these secrets—why shouldn't you?

Incidentally, you have my full permission to break any rules set down here. As long as you recognize their wisdom and break them *with style,* I'll be a happy camper.

> *I think it's very important to use fashion only as it serves you and not to become a slave of fashion. I think what's different now is that fashion is not so dictatorial anymore. There used to be a much stricter notion of what was appropriate to wear.*
>
> —PALOMA PICASSO, designer

1

THE TEN TOP REASONS FOR CAMOUFLAGE CHIC

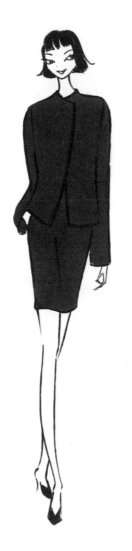

To look great, you have to be able to lethally assess your body and acknowledge the good and the bad bits.

—ELIZABETH HURLEY, actress/model/producer

1: WE ALL HAVE A LITTLE SOMETHING TO HIDE

No matter what dress size you are or how much you weigh, perfect proportions are hard to come by. Yes, there's always some little thing about us (or some big thing, for that matter) that keeps us humble and provides a sartorial challenge. That something can come in the form of superfluous bulges such as the ever-popular potbelly, a balance discrepancy such as a big hip/small rib cage combo, or a proportional variance—big legs, sloping shoulders, or short stature, for example.

One of my clients, for instance, has an arm thing. She's a size eight but has very long arms in relation to the rest of her body. She calls them monkey arms, which, being a wildlife enthusiast, I find rather charming. Before we had our first official wardrobe consultation, she had been buying clothes to fit her arms, which, not surprisingly, meant that the clothes were too big for the rest of her. She ended up looking lost in her oversized boxy business suits—and much less sleek and chic than she should have. Who would have guessed that a few extra inches in arm length could make such a difference to an entire look?

Let's face it, supermodels get the big bucks because, for whatever karmic reasons, they got blessed with near-perfect proportions, not to mention the impossibly photogenic faces. When they do have any proportional oddities, they are usually ones that work *for* them, not *against* them. That is, the disproportions make for an even taller and slimmer look. Take Nadja Auermann, for example. She's the German, usually platinum blond model who was dubbed "Der Stork" by her insensitive playmates as she was growing up. The moniker may have wounded her to the core as a child, but today she's cashing in big time on her remarkably long legs, which are a definite plus when it comes to wearing clothes well. So are long necks like Iman's . . . But enough about supermodels and their serendipitous oddities.

Most of us will find that our figure challenges are usually a little less advantageous than Der Stork's. And while Linda and Naomi, or Shalom and Amber, might look perfectly slim and adorable in an old tablecloth cinched in with a clothesline, the rest of us have to choose our outfits a little more carefully. We have to be totally aware of what we wear and how it affects our individual proportions. So take heed: We cannot wear *all* the stuff we see in magazines and expect to look just like the pictures. The women wearing those outfits are practically six feet tall and megaskinny. The average American woman is five feet, four inches tall and weighs 144 pounds. We need to think camouflage.

> *See perfection as a standard and imperfection as unique, singular, original. See it as the definition of you—the one and only you.*
>
> —ISABELLA ROSSELLINI, actress

2: THIS IS THE AGE OF SVELTE

Back in seventeenth-century Antwerp, Rubens's hefty models were considered perfect specimens of feminine pulchritude—veritable hot tomatoes, if you will. Today those very same women would be slurping Slim-Fast and pumping the StairMaster double time just to stay in business.

These days, looking slim is not just fashionable, it's a national obsession. Consider the run on fen-phen (when it was legal), the popularity of liposuction, the number of blockbuster diet books, the prevalence of low-fat snacks, low-cal food, diet drinks, and liquid food substitutes, the profitability of slim and trim gadgets like Thighmasters and Butt Busters, the profusion of weight reduction salons and overeaters' support groups, and the pervasiveness of eating disorders. Whew! The only thing Americans seem more obsessed with than looking thin is . . . *food!*

So if you care in the least about looking sleek and slender, you're in excellent company. You'd have to be living on another planet not to get caught up in the collective obsession. We have all, to one degree or another, bought into the ideal of svelte. It's a cultural thing—we can't avoid it. Until America as a whole starts embracing the full figure as the womanly ideal of beauty (as some other cul-

tures do), the pressure will be on to conform to one degree or another.

So my feeling is this: If you can't lick 'em, join 'em—not wholeheartedly, of course. I mean certainly not at the risk of your health. Go hook, line, and hold the sinker. Eat and exercise sensibly to stay within a range that's healthy and comfortable for your body, and *let your clothes take care of the rest.* Let us not forget that happiness is more important than a wispy waistline. If we're smart, our real personal goals will be more in the realm of total well-being—physical, mental, and spiritual. **On the**

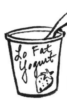

other hand, we all have to wear clothes, so we might as well follow the Rules of Camouflage Chic and pick ones that will give us an edge in the society of slim.

I don't believe that it's everybody to be a size eight or even a size twelve, I think you need to be where you physically feel the best for you.

—OPRAH WINFREY, talk show host etc.

3: UNLIKE SURGERY, CAMOUFLAGE DOESN'T HURT!

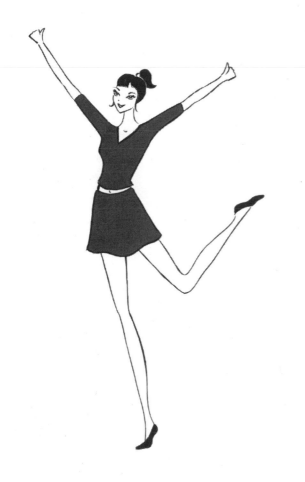

it to say, Camouflage Chic is a much milder, less perilous alternative—just a little harmless shopping with no recovery time. So forget that "No pain, no gain" mantra. It's old hat. The most agonizing part of Camouflage Chic is coming to grips with your imperfections. And since nobody else is perfect, that shouldn't be a big deal either. We're all in this together.

This is not to say, incidentally, that I'm not 110 percent in favor of exercise and good healthy eating habits. I'm not letting you off that easy. They're both too important for your well-being for you to ignore them. Although I'm no fitness guru, I do try to work out, eat well, and keep up. And study after study confirms that regular exercise and healthy eating habits decrease the risk of serious disease, increase longevity, and improve general health. And they give a very lovely natural glow, too. So let's hop to it!

Glamour was never my game. I just hate that thing about beauty. There's always someone out there better looking or worse looking. Beauty and glamour are not real things. To depend on them is very hard for anyone, but particularly hard for attractive girls.

—GENA ROWLANDS, actress

I don't think about being beautiful. What I devote most of my time to is being healthy.

—ANNE BANCROFT, actress

Camouflage Chic is the safest and the most painless way I know to look thinner. I'm too squeamish to get into the unappetizing details of liposuction—or the gruesome horror stories of overzealous or underqualified doctors, for that matter. And I'm sure you're aware of potential risks of diet drugs. Suffice

4: CAMOUFLAGE CHIC HELPS BOOST CONFIDENCE

I have heard with admiring submission the experience of the lady who declared that the sense of being perfectly well dressed gives a feeling of inward tranquility which religion is powerless to bestow.

—RALPH WALDO EMERSON,
essayist, poet, philosopher

Most of us feel better about ourselves when we're at our slimmest and know we look good to others. That's when we feel and exude the most self-confidence. I'm not saying that's how it should be, I'm just telling it like it is.

It's a part of the cultural thing that we discussed. Thanks to societal conditioning, a lot of us base a good part of our self-image on what others think of the size and shape of our bodies. We've been programmed that way since day one. Everywhere we look, we see that physical perfection begets praise, attention, fame, fortune, and frequently a rich husband—though not necessarily in that order. From Cinderella to Melrose Place, slim beauties win the day.

The early days, I think I looked better than I thought I did. . . . So now when I have a day when I feel unattractive, I say five years from now I'm gonna see a picture of myself and go, "I looked good!" It's just a mental thing.

—PAM TILLIS, singer

According to *The Body Project,* a fascinating look at the historical roots of our preoccupation with body size by Cornell professor Joan Jacobs Brumberg, fully 53 percent of American girls are unhappy with their bodies, and by the time they reach seventeen the number jumps to a whopping 78 percent. It's sad but, to some degree, fixable.

Dressing well can actually counterbalance some of that early programming and make us happier with our bodies. It can help build self-esteem, improve self-image, and boost sagging confidence. It's pretty simple psychology: You wear totally flattering clothes, you look in the mirror, you like what you see, and your spirits pick up.

To my mind, the Rules of Camouflage Chic give you the peace of mind to get you one step closer to where you want to be, which is feeling your best in any situation. Now, of course, body shape and size are only a *part* of your total appearance, not the whole enchilada. Certainly your attitudes, intelligence, manners, sparkle, grooming, et al. contribute significantly to the total package. Something seemingly as small as a dazzling smile can give you a big edge over some *über*-goddess. What you weren't given in height, you can make up for in grace. And what you didn't get in terms of bodily perfection, you can get by dressing cleverly to accentuate your positives and de-emphasize the negatives.

The secret of beauty is smiling and feeling good in yourself.

—SOPHIE MARCEAU, actress

5: FIRST IMPRESSIONS *DO* COUNT!

> *My mother ran the first store in Eugene, Oregon, that sold Birkenstocks. So you can understand my beauty problem. I grew up surrounded by hairy legs and sandals.*
>
> —COURTNEY LOVE, reformed grunge rocker

Before anybody gives you points for inner beauty or intellectual capacities, before they listen to your theories on cold fusion, global warming, or the necessity of zero population growth, they will—consciously or subconsciously—judge you by your appearance. According to statistics, more than half of a first impression is based on looks and demeanor. Most of the rest is based on speech qualities—whether you sound Park Avenue or trailer park. What you *actually* have to say counts for as little as 7 percent (which is why, I suppose, Cindy Crawford makes more money than Stephen Hawking).

Obviously, then, would it not behoove us to highlight our finest features and downplay our less luminous ones? Ideally, during a first glance, which usually lasts less than three seconds, you want your overall chic appearance to register first, followed, in short order, by your radiant face, which is your magnetic center of communication—unless, of course, you're Pamela Anderson Lee and have gone to considerable trouble and expense to focus the attention elsewhere.

Yes, you may, in fact, want to highlight other attractive features—great legs if you have them, or beautiful shoulders perhaps. But whatever your physical assets, the point is—and this is important—*they should be perceived first as part of the whole fabulous look, not as a separate body part.* And the same goes for less attractive features—they should be stylishly incorporated into the whole, not stand out on their own. There's no sense in allowing a bodily characteristic to leave the *first* memorable impression. Why be remembered as "the woman with the large behind" or "the babe with the big boobs"? The Rules of Camouflage Chic keep the attention focused where it should be—on the whole you, not just on your individual body parts. The Rules render any problem areas you might have less consequential.

> *I'm very broad-shouldered, long-armed like a gorilla.*
>
> —KATHARINE HEPBURN, actress

6: YOUR CLOTHES TALK—AND LOUDLY!

> *What you wear is a little story about your life.*
>
> —VICTORIA GALLEGOS, Prada supersaleswoman

Your clothes don't just talk about you, they practically scream—about everything from your socioeconomic status, taste, and character to your self-image, attitudes, and personality. They always have and they always will. Admittedly today's sartorial cues are more subtle than, say, in feudal times, when the aristocracy donned silks and the peasants huddled in unbleached homespun, but they're definitely still there for all to see. These cues have to do not only with the clothes you choose but how they fit, how you coordinate them, and how you accessorize them. A simple little black sheath, for instance, says something very different when it's perfectly tailored and worn with classy pumps and pearls than it does when it's skin tight and worn with fishnet stockings and stilettos.

The tenets of this book keep you in the "classy pumps" arena. They guarantee excellent nonverbal communication. The well-balanced, put-together proportions they propound suggest a balanced "together" mind-set—always a plus in personal and professional life. When you go by the Rules of Camouflage Chic, the messages you send are ones of elegance, savvy, confidence, and sophistication. You never feel insecure or look as if you're trying to prove anything. Your clothes say, "I don't have to try to look good—I just do." So what if your unstudied elegance is a just a tad studied? Who has to know? As Jackie Mason would say, "So what is that their business?"

> *I put Tony in muted dense dyes and in soft-to-the-touch fabrics. I also put him in crêpes. Crêpe drapes fabulously. It's a sexy fabric. I wanted to help him convey that he was stylish—of the moment, young, open to change. More than anything else, friendly. Crêpe communicated his personality—the boy next door, so normal. Except he isn't.*
>
> —MALCOLM LEVENE, British designer/tailor/image maker, on dressing British Prime Minister Tony Blair

7: BECAUSE YOU MIGHT BE VERTICALLY CHALLENGED

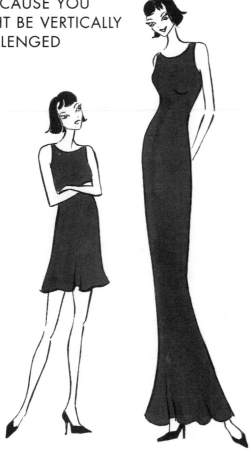

I mention it here only as a reason for Camouflage Chic because when you're short, as I'm sure anybody under five-three has noticed, every extra pesky ounce shows threefold. There simply isn't as much body space for extra weight to be distributed. A five-foot, nine-inch woman has plenty of area over which to disperse a few extra pounds. Most of the rest of us don't. For the same reason, things like long and short waists, big busts, wide hips, etc., are more obvious on short women. So if you're a tad undersized, *elongation through fashion* is especially important, which makes the upcoming rules a natural, since elongation is one of our main goals.

Another thing that short women have to consider is *scale*, which as you know is the size of something in relation to something else. Since a short woman has a smaller fashion canvas to work with—that is, less actual space to cover with clothing and accessories—she has to keep her fashion relatively uncluttered and scale appropriate. This means that details such as lapels, pockets, buttons, prints, patterns, etc. generally need to be smaller. Something as simple as oversize jacket lapels can throw her entire look totally out of balance—and we discuss that here, too. In other words, all the Rules of Camouflage Chic are totally applicable to small women!

I'm so small, so if clothes have too many buttons or pockets or color schemes I get lost in them.

—PRISCILLA PRESLEY, actress

I'm short so I need a little lift, but I'm not comfortable with a three-and-a-half-inch spike heel.

—GERALDINE FERRARO, politician

First, I have to point out that unless you have serious professional basketball or supermodel aspirations, there is absolutely nothing wrong with being short. Short can be chic. My aunt Rose is short and she is perfectly adorable. Since, as previously mentioned, the average American woman is five feet, four inches tall, *short-ish* is actually the norm.

8: BECAUSE YOU MIGHT BE A FULL-FIGURED GAL

> *Having curves and hips is a lot easier than try-ing to achieve that old-school elegant, willowy look. I hope the larger look stays because then I can keep eating my fried chicken.*
>
> —JENNIFER TILLY, **actress**

Full-figured means "busty" for all you gals who are too young to re-member that old Jane Russell Playtex bra commercial. Big breasts come and go. They were *démodé* in the Roar-ing Twenties, when flat-chested flappers were the rage, back in vogue big time in the fifties, when Jane and her pal Marilyn Monroe were in their prime, out of style again in the sixties, when Twiggy was the It Girl . . . and now? Well, now they're quite acceptable really, and even semidesirable, but definitely not a must-have item. Some models have them, some don't, and movie stars like Meg Ryan, Cameron Diaz, and Gwyneth Paltrow seem to be doing just fine without them. There's that timing thing again.

The thing about big breasts, be they natural or man-made, is that they add dimension, and that dimension has to blend gracefully with the rest of your proportions. If you're tall and fairly evenly proportioned, they can look wonderful—curvy, feminine, and sexy. On the other hand, if you're short, short-waisted, or plump all over, the extra dimension tends to dominate your whole upper body and can make you look boxy and chunky in clothes, which, heaven forbid, can trans-late as matronly.

By the way, **big hips** are often another part of being a full-figured gal that Ms. Jane Russell forgot to mention. They're probably the most common fe-male figure challenge going—like love handles for men, only harder to cover up and not as charitably accepted. In and of themselves, full hips are actu-ally not a problem. If you were six feet tall and had full hips and full everything else, you could be a sexy Amazon goddess—full-figured, but well bal-anced. But as we know, five-foot-four is the norm, so kiss that fantasy good-bye. Most big hips—whether they're matched with a smallish rib cage, which makes for your prototypical pear shape, or with a full bosom and wasp waist à la your classic Gibson girl—can benefit from tender loving cam-ouflage. And we'll get to that a little later.

> *In order to know what works well on your body you have to be comfortable with it. That's the grail.*
>
> —MINNIE DRIVER, **actress**

9: YIKES! BAT WINGS, BELLY ROLLS, BANANA ROLLS, AND THUNDER THIGHS

> *You have to remember there are some things in life more important than fabulous thighs.*
>
> —WYNONNA JUDD, singer

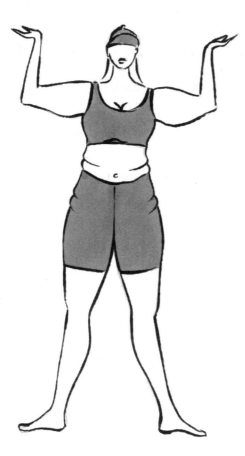

"Bat wings, belly rolls, banana rolls, and thunder thighs" are not an assortment of exotic hors d'oeuvres. They are a collection of hard-hearted, callous terms for some of our pesky little figure challenges. They were probably thought up by some shlump with serious mother issues, so you can't really take them seriously. On the other hand, you might want to have at least a passing familiarity with these slights, just in case you hear them being bandied about on *Jerry Springer* or *Ricki Lake*.

Bat wings are those little jiggly areas of loose flesh that some women have hanging from their upper arms—often the result of excess weight or age, or even genetics. Truly, nobody's immune. A while back, even American icon Kathie Lee Gifford discovered her own personal set—a fact she generously shared with her TV audience. Kathie Lee jokingly jiggled her bat wings for the entire world, then booked a triceps exercise specialist for the show the next day. Triceps exercises are actually a good preventative measure, but if you already have bat wings, they're hard to shake—well, actually easy to shake, hard to get rid of. So your best bet is to 1. be grateful that you have arms that work at all, then 2. camouflage them. Same thing for heavy arms in general (see page 52).

Belly rolls are the result of that extra layer of padding that somehow seems to find its way to your stomach and the area just above it, where it adheres like Krazy Glue. When you bend over, the flesh tends to *roll*, hence the name. While they may sound cute and jolly, they're actually rather unsettling when they appear out of nowhere—usually just after the Thanksgiving and Christmas holidays and/or when you've just been invited to a pool party. Even one little belly roll, singular, is enough to unravel a former hard body. Still, all in all, they're relatively innocuous from a Camouflage Chic point of view—very easy to disguise.

Banana rolls. If you're not fond of belly rolls, you probably won't be thrilled with banana rolls either—once you know about them, anyway. Actually, I have to admit this is a new one on me, too. Banana rolls, apparently, are those extra strips of flesh women get just below their buttocks. Who knew? Again, though, they are simply a minor annoyance, not particularly hazardous to one's sartorial health. The best idea is probably just not to look at your backside for too long in a full-length mirror. Problem solved.

Thunder thighs. I don't know why I find this one particularly grating; it's no more malicious than the rest. Maybe it annoys me because I've actually heard mean little kids taunting their playmates with it. Karma will take care of them in their forties. Anyway, thunder thighs are simply large thighs. Nothing to worry about, really. Besides, what's large in one context is small in another. Garden-variety thunder thighs pale in comparison to those amazing colorful spandexed specimens on the speed-skating rinks at the Winter Olympics. Weren't they a wonder to behold? Maybe big thighs are on their way to becoming fashionable! Meanwhile, we'll just whittle them away with our Camouflage Chic techniques.

There are probably scads of other terms like the above floating around the universe. But the final caveat here is never, ever take them to heart. They are *truly inconsequential* in the cosmic scheme of things. Simply tuck your copy of *Does This Make Me Look Fat?* under your arm, throw your head back, and laugh like a debutante.

> *I've always had a curvaceous body. But I've [also] always had a big butt.*
>
> —JENNIFER LOPEZ, actress

10: CAMOUFLAGE CHIC— BECAUSE YOU CAN!

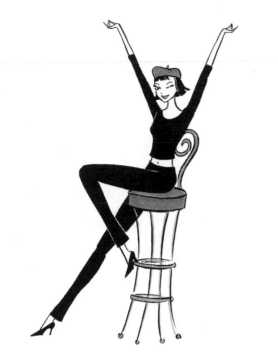

tage of them? Plus, Camouflage Chic provides something we need but don't readily get from today's fashion industry—a yardstick by which we can measure our fashion decisions. Much of the clothing we see on the runways and in the magazines is more art than anything else—conceptual, inspirational, and even political. It's not altogether wearable. So even if we had the figures to wear the whimsical alluring designs, would we? Where would we go in them? How would they fit into our lifestyles?

> *Haute couture should be fun, foolish, and almost unwearable.*
>
> —CHRISTIAN LACROIX, designer

> *Confidence, darling, is elegance.*
>
> —DESIREE MEJER, designer

The last and probably most compelling reason of all to go the Camouflage Chic route is because *there's no reason not to.* The rules are all here to help make you look great. Why not take advan-

Since we can't follow the fashion pages per se, it's up to us to design our own wardrobes for ourselves. We have to go into the stores and pick and choose and put things together that work for our individual bodies. The upcoming Rules make that easier. They take the guesswork out of shopping and give you a nice solid foundation to build on . . . so here we go!

2

THE DEFINITIVE RULES
OF CAMOUFLAGE CHIC

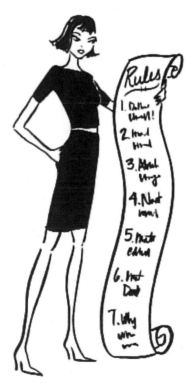

Most women are not aware of their beauty, they're most aware of their defects.

—FREDERIC FEKKAI, hair guru

The following pearls of wisdom are based on the fact that every piece of clothing you put on your body is made up of four basic design elements: proportion, line, color, and texture. To look your slimmest, each of those elements has to be right on target—and perfectly in sync with your body. These rules show you how to hit the bull's-eye on all accounts. So without further ado . . .

RULE 1

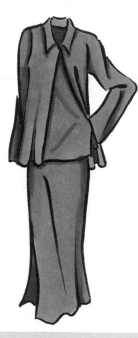

MONOCHROMATIC IS MAGIC!

> Color is like food for the spirit—plus it's not addictive or fattening.
>
> —ISAAC MIZRAHI, designer

Monochromatic dressing is the favorite trick of virtually every fashion editor, designer, and stylist I know. Even Giorgio Armani and Donna Karan are adherents in their personal lives. Why? Because it makes everybody look slimmer and taller instantly. Plus, it's always elegant, and it's an extremely easy way to dress—almost a total no-brainer! You have to wonder why more women outside the fashion industry don't take advantage of it.

Technically, dressing monochromatically is wearing one color—any color—from head to toe (although we can fudge that bit, as you'll see in a minute), and it works for two main reasons. *Number one, color is the first thing most people notice about an outfit.* Even someone who is clueless about fashion and rarely notices what anybody's wearing will notice color. And *number two, dressing in one color produces a strong unbroken vertical line that elongates the body.* Put those two facts together and you've got **a very powerful slimming tool.**

Audrey Hepburn was one of the multitude of stylish celebrities who fully appreciated the marvels of monochromes. There's the much-told story of how Audrey was driven to tears during the making of *Funny Face* by director Stanley Donen's insistence that she wear white socks with her black dancer's outfit. Audrey tried to explain that the socks would interrupt the continuous black line of her outfit and make her legs look shorter, but Donen, apparently unschooled in the finer nuances of Camouflage Chic, just didn't get it. Ultimately, Audrey wore the maligned socks and after seeing the footage actually acknowledged that in that particular cinematic instance they were, in fact, acceptable, since they helped to separate her from the background. I don't think she ever incorporated the socks into her personal wardrobe, however.

> What I love about fashion is it is an expression of personality. What I hate about fashion is anything forced.
>
> —KELLY KLEIN, photographer

Use Texture to Add Interest to Monochromes

While we're talking one color here, we're in no way limiting texture. You can incorporate as many different textures into an outfit as you like—within reason, of course (see Rule 7 for restrictions). In fact, you'd be surprised at the extra pizzazz and sophistication you can get with a little warp and woof. Imagine the rich interplay of a buttery soft suede jacket, cashmere turtleneck, fluid wool flannel trousers, and silk scarf. Even if all the colors were identical, the variation in textures would give the outfit a rich, interesting dimension and relief from sameness.

With textures like ribbing, knits, tweeds, and jacquard-type fabrics, you can even add patterns without ever getting near another color. Plus, texture can even help define the mood of your outfit. You could, for instance, add a touch of affluence with

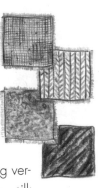

silk charmeuse, a hint of femininity with lace or chiffon, or a dash of romanticism with velvet. So take advantage of texture. It can lend as much interest and pizzazz as a second color but offers much less risk of leading the eye off its slimming vertical course. Try a navy silk charmeuse shell with your navy gabardine suit, for instance, or a wonderful navy chiffon and velvet scarf, or both.

> *Style is not something applied. It is something that permeates. It is of the nature of that in which it is found, whether the poem, the manner of a god, the bearing of a man. It is not a dress.*
>
> —WALLACE STEVENS, poet

How to Bend the Monochromatic Rule

Of course, you can bend the rule. You didn't think I was going to keep you in fashion jail, did you?

ALERT

These days, all the old rules about what fabrics you can or cannot mix have been tossed to the wind. Designers mix everything with anything, and so can you. Our only texture-mix taboos are those that may potentially add girth, so please see Rule 7 before mixing satin hot pants with your leather motorcycle jacket.

There will probably be times when you just don't *feel* like dressing in one color. Even I, who have more black in my closet than a nun, occasionally get the urge to mix and match a color or two—not often, mind you, but it does happen. So a little cheating is fine, as long as we don't lose the monochromatic magic. Once we start on this course, the resulting outfits might not be *technically* monochromatic, but they'll be real close, which is good enough. Bending a rule is always fun if you can get away with it.

> *I usually wear one color. I'm only five-foot four; one color makes me look taller and thinner—which is always good for the camera and my own self-esteem.*
>
> —MING-NA WEN, actress

PLAY AROUND WITH VALUES

The first bend in the road is the **juxtaposition of values.** *Value* is the lightness or darkness of a color. Black is the darkest value, white the lightest. Every other color falls somewhere in between. It's really easy to see value when you look at black and white photographs because it's the only color element that actually comes through. Medium red and medium green, for instance, come across as the same shade of gray. Ditto for pale yellow and pale pink, or dark brown and navy. So when you're trying to determine the value of a particular color, just imagine what shade of gray it would be in a black-and-white photograph. The closer the shades of gray, the closer the colors are in value.

One value of different colors: Theoretically, you could mix almost any colors of the same value and create some pretty spiffy fashion combinations. In the pastel ranges, for instance, you could mix a yummy mélange of dusty pinks and blues, lavenders, muted greens, and melons. Bright combos such as red and purple, bright blue and emerald, turquoise and yellow might also be viable and exciting. *But if you're serious about looking thinner your best bet is to mix subtle dark colors,* such as navy and deep loden green, mink brown and charcoal gray, deep wine and raisin, or any of the above with black. It's a very effective and creative way to skirt the monochromatic rule. The slight variations in color add interest, but you get almost the same solidarity as a single color since the eye is not terribly distracted. It works best with the darker tones because they absorb light and seem to blend seamlessly together. The intensity of the brighter colors, on the other hand, tends to draw the eye to where the two colors meet, which would be risky in terms of camouflage if the colors intersected in an undesirable area, say across the hips. Not only would you be drawing attention to where you might not want it, but a horizontal line would be created that would interrupt the vertical line of the body.

One color of different values: The other value-mixing tactic is to **blend different values of the same color.** In other words, blend lighter and darker shades of one color. You could blend a range of grays, for instance, from pearl to putty to slate to charcoal, or a palette of browns from taupe to cocoa to chocolate. **It's always a good idea to keep lighter tones on top for balance.** Also, since lighter tones draw attention first, they lead the eye up to your lovely face and away from any potential trouble spots. Blends in the same color family give the impression of solid color unity and make for a longer and leaner look. Plus, they are quite chic and very sophisticated to boot.

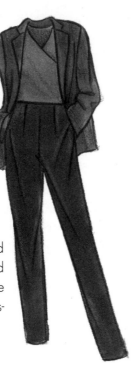

> *Color should please the eye, not overwhelm it, and enhance the physicality of the person who wears it.*
>
> —Vivienne Tam, designer

SLIP IN A TEENY BIT OF A SECOND COLOR

The last loophole in the monochromatic rule is to introduce a *relatively* small amount of a second unrelated color of your choice. I suppose this dodge could be technically termed dichromatic, but let's not get nitpicky. I think of the second color as your *uplift color,* because that's what it should do—pick up your spirits, warm your skin, and add glow. Camel and pea green, then, would not be good uplift colors. **The trick is to keep your base color dominant and use your uplift color sparingly.** A reasonable ratio would be base color 75 percent, uplift color 25 percent or even less.

Then consider **placement:** Where you put that colorful 25 percent is significant. There are essentially two major places it can go: on the *inside* of the silhouette or on the *outside.* Let's talk about the inside first.

Add color on the inside with tops, scarves, and jewelry: Plan one requires a second layer such as a jacket or cardigan. Keep the **outer silhouette (say, a suit) one solid color and introduce your uplift color on the inside** in the form of tops: blouses, vests, sweaters, and scarves. (No bright sashes around hips or waist, please—see Rule 3.) If you were wearing a black suit, for instance, you could wear a colorful print scarf or a brightly colored blouse—anything from yellow to periwinkle to red—*under* the jacket. Whatever color you chose, you'd still reap some of the benefits of monochrome because the *outer* silhouette would still be one color and would still be producing a strong vertical color line. Would you look as skinny as you would dressed in one solid color from top to bottom? Yes, if the uplift color is mainly up around your neck—as it would be with a scarf, or a collar peeking out of a *closed* jacket. You would probably not look quite as thin with a colored top interrupting the line. But you would still be in very acceptable CC territory.

Rosie O'Donnell dresses the first way a lot on her show. That is, she'll wear a dark pantsuit with a brightly colored shirt—the collar of which, more often than not, comes out over the lapels. I've heard some snooty fashion critics rag Rosie for not being a little more adventurous, but I say give the girl some slack. She's doing just great—especially from a camouflage point of view. The monochromatic suit is slimming; the flash of color at the neck keeps the look interesting enough for TV; she always looks comfortable because the whole look suits her personality; and, best of all, the strongest impression is simply that Rosie looks good. Your focus is on *her,* more than what she's wearing or the shape of her body. Even though Rosie is a big woman, she never looks particularly fat, which makes her a winner in my book. Frankly, I'd hate to see what some of those critics would put her in.

Other ways to add color: There are lots of variations on this theme. For example, black pants paired with a black V-neck sweater over a white or colored T-shirt is a great casual look. The V neck allows you to add color easily without disturbing the overall monochrome. You get the same effect with dark leggings and a longish V-neck tunic (in the same

color) worn over a T-shirt, turtleneck, or banded-neck collar. It's all the same principle.

Other necklines can work too. You could wear one scoop-neck top over another, for instance, letting the colorful one underneath peek out a bit. I wear double tank tops all the time in summer—usually white over black or black over white. I get a little extra coverage and a little extra zip. Basically, no matter what shape the neckline, it's all the same idea: *A brighter or contrasting color near your face draws the attention up and adds interest to the outfit.* We love that! (Also see Rule 10.)

Add color with jackets: Plan two: While Rosie adds her color to the inside of her outfit, the opposite approach is also valid—although a tad riskier: **Keep the inner silhouette totally monochromatic and add a second color to the outer one.** You could, for example, wear a bright blazer with your black turtleneck and slacks. (Although, unless you're a Washington politico, I personally would prefer to see you in the more subtle shades.) You'd be on the outer limits of our 75/25 percent rule, if not stepping over it, but as long as your core outfit is a dark monochrome, **you'll still look relatively thin because you'll be creating a strong dark vertical line of color straight down the middle of your body.** The eye will interpret the long dark vertical as your skinny silhouette.

You could take the idea even further to very dramatic effect with a striking or exotic coat over a dark inner core. Here the *inner* silhouette color becomes 25 percent of the ensemble and the coat becomes the 75 percent. One of my style-conscious friends enthuses that Kim Novak has never looked as slim and trim as she did in *Vertigo* when she was wearing her memorable heavy white coat/diaphanous black dress ensemble. I've also seen pictures of Marlene Dietrich looking equally svelte in her version of the same. When it works, it works, I guess. But I still hesitate to endorse the look for us regular folks. The cut of the coat would have to be *exquisite*—and think of the cleaning bills!

The key thing to remember when mixing disparate colors is to *always avoid stark color contrasts in places that will divide the body into two distinct sections.* A body divided is a shorter and heavier body. A white blouse with a black skirt, for instance, divides the body right in half. But when you pop on a black jacket with it, you've got a strong monochromatic outer silhouette, a 75/25 percent color ratio, and voilà, you *are* Camouflage Chic.

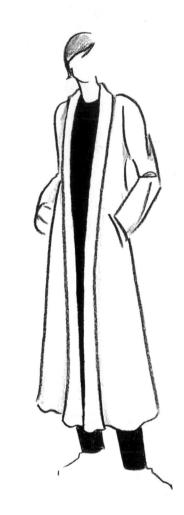

> To look your slimmest when dealing with two colors, keep one color dominant. Aim for a ratio of 75 percent one color to 25 percent the other.

RULE 2

BASE YOUR WARDROBE ON DARK NEUTRALS

> *With a black pullover and ten rows of pearls, she revolutionized fashion.*
>
> —CHRISTIAN DIOR, designer, on Coco Chanel

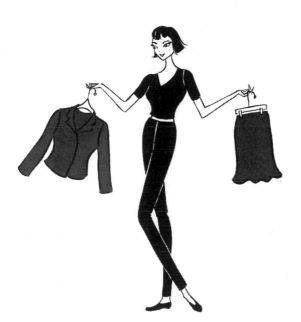

You may have noticed that the majority of the examples in Rule 1 feature dark or darkish neutrals. It wasn't by accident. Although the monochromatic plan will work in every color of the rainbow, *dark neutral colors make you look thinnest.* That's just the way it is. They may not be the most exhilarating colors, or the most romantic, or the most adventurous, but they are the most slimming. And they're chic, sophisticated, and versatile, to boot.

The secret behind the slimming power of darker colors is their ability to absorb light and recede into the background—rather than reflect light and pop out, as lighter and brighter colors do. Plus, extraneous details and construction lines, such as seams and darts, are absorbed by the *density* of dark colors, leaving fewer lines to distract the eye. Think of any of the pale blouses in your closet. In most, you can probably see outlines of seam allowances, shoulder pads, and sometimes underwear. Not so with dark colors. **The darker the color, the more invisible the construction.** Which, incidentally, is why it's easier to get away with dark inexpensive garments. Even fabric quality is less discernible.

Darker colors are also kinder on lumps and bumps. The other day I noticed a heavyish woman in a light seafoam green tunic top and matching tights. She had a bad case of cellulite on her thighs, which showed right through the tights. Had she been wearing a dark color that absorbed the light rather than reflected it, the bumps would have practically disappeared. If only she'd asked . . .

Fashion Neutrals

A good fashion neutral is a color that is not trendy, is easy to mix and match, complements your skin tone, and blends well with other colors you like to wear. A good darkish fashion neutral has all those attributes and is medium to dark toned in color. Lime green and tangerine obviously don't cut the mustard. (Nor does mustard, come to think of it.) Creams and beiges are terrific neutrals and can be wonderfully chic but are too light in tone to make the surefire Camouflage Chic list. Navy and black are perfect Camouflage Chic dark neutrals. **The darker the color, the safer you are.**

Black Magic

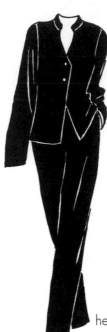

> *Black is the essential uniform. It takes you from day to evening. It's always safe . . . and it's always sexy. . . . For myself, I feel thinner in black.*
>
> —DONNA KARAN, designer

Black, in fact, is the prima, number one, best dark fashion neutral of all time and will be for ever and ever—for the following reasons: First, it's the most slimming color on the planet. And from there it just gets better: It goes with just about every other color imaginable or stands proudly by itself. It's chic for daytime and evening; perfect for almost any occasion; looks rich; is cross-seasonal; will never go out of style; conceals dirt, thus requiring less maintenance; is inconspicuous enough to be worn fre-

quently without anyone noticing it. Plus, it's a great backdrop for jewelry.

> *Black is the power color. Black is chic, severe, and it shows off your jewelry better.*
>
> —NANCY COLLINS, journalist

I confess—no big surprise here—that I'm a practicing dyed-in-the-wool blackaholic. I did my color thing in the seventies. Now I'm more interested in ease, speed, and comfort—and black serves the purpose well. I open a closet full of black stuff, pull something out, everything goes with everything else, I don't look fat. It's heaven! But as addicted as I am personally, I wouldn't think of suggesting that everybody else wear black all the time—well, I might think of it, but I wouldn't do it. There's no reason we all have to look like Greek widows. On the other hand, if you're looking for a

---

HOW TO PERK UP YOUR BASIC BLACK

- Introduce textures with blouses, scarves, and shawls. Try sheers, crêpe, silk charmeuse, velvet, chiffon, etc.
- Add sparkle with jewelry. Silver, gold, pearls, diamonds, even minerals like jade and carnelian . . . everything looks great with black.
- Don't be afraid to mix with navy and browns.
- Wear your favorite colors around your face.
- For accents try cream or ivory instead of white for a more sophisticated look.

goof-proof, easy-to-manage wardrobe scheme, I do highly recommend that you **pick a darkish neutral or two that you like and that suit your skin tone and build your wardrobe around them.** You don't have to wear dark neutrals exclusively (although you'd look thinnest if you did); just make them the foundation of your wardrobe.

> *I wear black. Black is the safest thing. I never wear plaids. I hardly ever wear prints. My closet is really, really, really, really boring—mostly dark colors in there.*
>
> —REBA MCENTIRE, singer

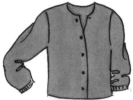

That means that the basic pieces of your wardrobe—your jackets, skirts, slacks, suits, and coats—should be in one or more dark neutral shades. If you choose more than one, the colors should blend flawlessly—say black and dark brown, or gray flannel and charcoal, for instance—so that you can always mix and match effectively. If you want to add snappier colors, you can always do it with blouses, sweaters, scarves, and other accessories.

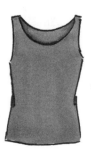

Just how many dark neutral basics you need in your wardrobe depends primarily on your pocketbook and how much variety you like in life. You could form a terrific working wardrobe based all on one dark neutral color (as I do), or you could put together

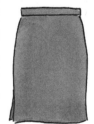

an equally terrific, but more diverse, wardrobe based on two or more neutrals. It's really more of a time/money/lifestyle decision than a fashion one. **The fewer colors in your closet, the simpler your fashion life.** More colors call for more shoes, bags, and other accessories—which means more shopping, more closet space, and more money.

So it's up to you. The easiest route? Start out with one of the tried-and-true dark neutrals, such as the aforementioned black, navy, deep chocolate brown, charcoal, gray flannel, or dark taupe, and gradually introduce other colors as you find special pieces you love.

> *Because black absorbs light, it shows the fewest imperfections. It recedes, but at the same time it outlines the shape of the body. When I design something new, I use black as my base.*
>
> —DONNA KARAN, designer

Although theoretically you could also build a splendid wardrobe based on more exotic dark colors, such as dark muted periwinkle, deep olive, aubergine, or any of the complex gray-browns, you'd find them considerably harder to match up and update over the years—as well as less versatile and trickier to accessorize. There will be new designs every year in black and navy. There may or may not be new designs in aubergine or periwinkle. **Bottom line: It will always be easier to** find wardrobe updates, additions, and matching accessories in classic colors. On the other hand, if you run in the same circles as Ivana Trump, a wardrobe full of fabulous exotic darkish colors is a perfectly viable alternative—just call your people and have them make up whatever you need.

Bonus Points for Dark Neutrals

A few more quick points on the glories of dark neutral colors before we move on. First, they are, for the most part, what I call *mood neutral*. They tend to let your personality and style shine through more than do other colors. Other colors can be rather chatty when you think about it. Pastels whisper feminine gentility, bright colors shout outgoing and fun, dull colors proclaim conservatism, and so on. If anything, dark colors might be conceived of as dramatic, but their overall effect is much more dependent on what you bring to them: how you wear them, where you wear them, and your personality. They become an almost integral part of you.

Second, dark neutrals are simply more appropriate for more occasions and have the added bonus of being very easy to dress up with accessories. And like black, other dark neutral colors are much less conspicuous than their brighter or lighter cousins—hence people notice them less, which

means you can wear them more often. All very handy in an office environment and for those of us with small closets. In the long run, dark neutrals simply give you a lot more bang for your buck.

> *You wear black and you don't compete with the environment. I don't think there's ever been a time when black has been so permanently a part of the color fabric.*
>
> —BETH ANN HARDISON, model manager

Exception: As I mentioned, cream and beige are *not* surefire slimmers, but you can get so many great sophisticated looks by blending different tones of the beige family that I just can't bring myself to rule them out absolutely. Yes, they are definitely way out of the "darkish" range, but I feel their rich, timeless chic compensates for their light color. (What can I say, sometimes I have to break even my own rules.) This is a good loophole, incidentally, for those of you in more tropical climes who might need to lighten up now and then. You could also try light grays and mix in more midtones if you like. Just stick to the strategies we discussed in Rule 1, and you should be just fine.

ISAAC MIZRAHI ON THE LITTLE BLACK DRESS

"I think it started when Eve was looking around for the perfect black fig leaf. But when I think of the little black dress, I think of Norell, who glorified it. I mean, that was what his whole career was about. I also think about Audrey Hepburn in *Breakfast at Tiffany's* living every single day in the same black dress with different accessories and making it look new every day. And I think about the woman in the nineties who needs to wear the same thing from eight in the morning until midnight."

RULE 3

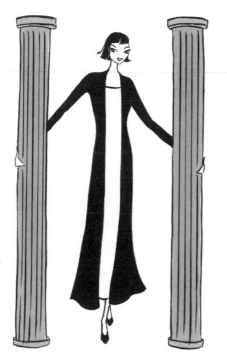

> You've got to know the shape of your body and accentuate what God gave you.
>
> —LELA ROCHON, actress

This is THE most important design rule going. So if you're sitting there sipping a diet cola thinking, Yeah, yeah, I know I'm not supposed to wear horizontal stripes, hang on a minute. Vertical lines in fashion are about a whole lot more than stripes—and even stripes are a tad trickier than you might think—so no flipping.

Aside from stripes, lines show up in all sorts of unexpected places: in a garment's cut and styling, its design detailing, fabric drape, silhouette, and color (as we've just discussed in Rules 1 and 2). **These kinds of lines are considerably more subtle than your garden-variety stripe,** and their signifi-

VERTICALS ARE YOUR FRIENDS

cance is easy to miss, but they can make a tremendous difference in terms of looking thinner.

How It Works

Vertical lines, as we all know, go up and down, as opposed to horizontal lines, which go side to side. *The basic theory is this: The faster the eye scans a line, the longer and narrower the area it defines will seem.* Since the eye scans vertical lines very quickly, your body will appear longer and narrower (taller and slimmer) when it's clothed in vertical lines. On the other hand, since the eye loves nothing more than resting on peaceful horizons, it follows horizontal lines very *slowly*. So you will appear *wider and shorter* in clothes with horizontal lines. And finally, because the eye also shifts into low gear when it follows curved lines, they can make you look larger as well.

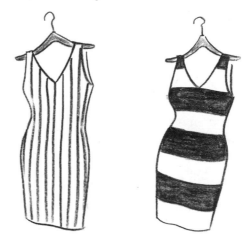

With that in mind, vertical lines are the indisputable winners in the Camouflage Chic sweepstakes. Of course, we'll always have to deal with some horizontal and curved lines since they are integral parts of both fashion and our bodies—hemlines and waistlines are intrinsic fashion horizontals; busts and shoulders are natural figure horizontals. **But for the most part, we'll always be on a quest for garments, outfits, and accessories that will reinforce strong vertical lines.** Before we go any further, though, let me get two minor vertical line exceptions out of the way. . . .

A Few *Unfriendly* Verticals!

Vertical stripes are the most obvious vertical lines in fashion. So theoretically they should help create a long slim look, but in some instances they can do just the opposite. They are, for one, **positively *deadly* on tight stretchy fabrics.**

I once bought a pair of gray pin-striped leggings. They were top quality *and* heavily discounted, so how could I resist? Big mistake. The

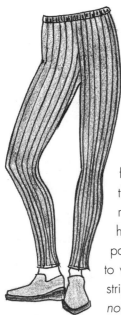

stripes, vertical though they were, curved right over my thighs, hips, and stomach, echoing every single little bulge and bump along the way! Ick! I wore them for about four minutes and quickly passed them along to a bulgeless, bumpless friend. The same frightening thing could happen with ribbed tights, striped panty hose, or even snug corduroy pants. So be warned: You have to watch how you wear vertical stripes, and one way definitely *not* to wear them is tight.

Also, **watch out for broad vertical stripes that are widely spaced.** When there's a lot of space between stripes, the eye is led side to side as well as up and down, which can leave you looking more wide than narrow. Other than these rather esoteric exceptions, vertical lines will elongate the body and make you look slimmer.

Diagonal Lines

Diagonal lines, which move the eye across the body at an angle, come in second place in our sweepstakes— *as long as the angle is more vertical than horizontal.* The steeper and more vertical the diagonal line, the more elongating it will be.

Horizontal Lines

Horizontal lines generally get a pretty bad "wrap" in fashion circles, and for the most part it's well deserved. Most horizontal lines are deadly. Some however, are less lethal than others—a thin horizontal seam is obviously going to take less of a toll than a wide colorful ruffle. And there are also one or two horizontal lines that are actually relatively benign.

The crucial differential between deadly and benign is **placement.** You have to keep horizontal lines away from areas that are wide to start with. A broad horizontal band across the hips, for instance, would be particularly disastrous on three accounts: 1. It would add a couple of virtual inches to the hips; 2. it would direct attention to the hips;

and 3. it would interrupt the vertical line of the body and visually shorten the legs. You would, in a word, look fat.

A horizontal higher up on the body, on the other hand, say between the bust and the waistline as per an Empire waist, would be less detrimental proportionately, since the legs would look longer, and, as I've mentioned, the longer your legs, the taller you'll look. (Warning: Empire-waist dresses lean toward the unsophisticated—choose wisely.)

In some cases, horizontal lines can, if cleverly placed, even help balance specific proportional discrepancies. If, for instance, you're a classic pear shape (wide below the waist and narrow above), horizontal lines across the shoulders and chest could broaden your torso a bit. But as you'll see in Rule 4, you must watch the balance very closely, lest you overcompensate and end up looking boxy and chunky. Even if you use horizontal lines to broaden your shoulders, **your *overall* outfit still has to be geared toward elongation to make you look your slimmest.**

I have this obsession with lines. Like on a Rodin sculpture, the lines of clothes have to be fluid and highlight your best attributes. I don't like clothes that are confining and interrupt those lines. Giorgio Armani knows what I'm talking about.

—Johnathon Schaech, actor

Putting Theory into Practice

As I mentioned, both dreaded horizontal lines and helpful vertical lines show up in very subtle little places: pockets, seams and darts, buttons and other closures, necklines, fabric drapes and folds, color, and design. The following sketches will help you recognize them and decide which ones to embrace and which to avoid.

THE BOTTOM LINE ON LINES

Consciously look to create verticals. Keep a sharp eye on horizontals—don't let them be the dominant lines in any outfit, and whatever you do, never wear them across your widest point—especially your hips and derriere.

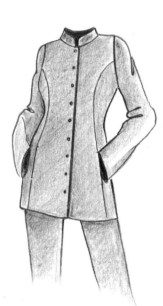

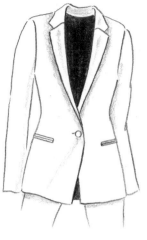

The narrow lapels of this classic-cut jacket create flattering diagonal lines. Because the armhole is relatively high, there is a long, lean vertical line from armpit to the jacket hem, and the sleeves are narrow.

Camouflage Chic Rating: A

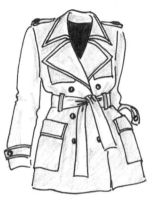

There are mostly friendly verticals here. The narrow cut and monochromatic color scheme create a lovely vertical silhouette, with no horizontal interruptions. Even the pockets are cleverly hidden in *vertical* seams, a real plus. The line of buttons down the front of the jacket adds another vertical line. Ditto for the mandarin collar.

Camouflage Chic Rating: A+

This safari look is a triple threat: too many horizontal lines created by too many pockets. Plus, the belt breaks the vertical line of the jacket at the waist, and the collar is way too wide.

Camouflage Chic Rating: F

The contoured silhouette of this fitted suit is good, but the lighter-toned hip pockets and round lapels keep it from being a total winner. See how much slimmer it looks with less curved, less contrasting lapels and *no* hip pockets.

Camouflage Chic Rating: C

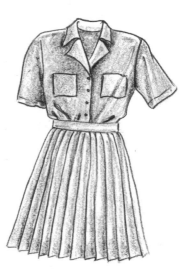

The skirt is too stiff, with no real drape or movement. So instead of falling into pleasing verticals, it stands alone as one solid fat-making block. The wide boat-neck collar and hip band on the sweater add unnecessary horizontals.

Camouflage Chic Rating: D

The pleats on this skirt form verticals, but there are too many of them. The eye jumps from side to side across them, instead of following them up and down, and all the benefits of the vertical lines are lost. The patch pockets on the blouse also lead the eye from side to side, further complicating the issue.

Camouflage Chic Rating: F

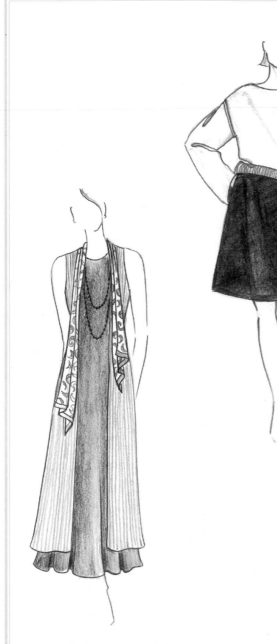

Here, vertical lines are created by the soft drape of the skirt and the long, narrowly cut knit vest. The long silk scarf and beads reinforce the verticals another degree.

Camouflage Chic Rating: B

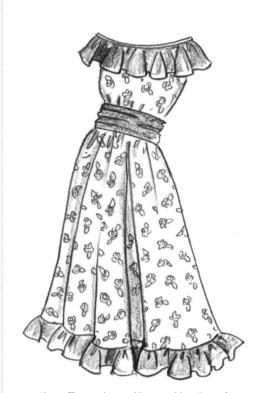

The ruffles at the neckline and hemline of this questionably designed frock form two disastrous fluffy horizontal lines. The sash at the waist adds insult to injury. Nobody stands a chance in this horizontal chaos.

Camouflage Chic Rating: **F–**

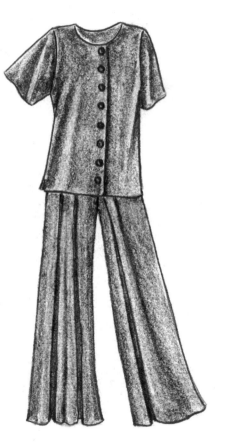

The ultrawide leg on these palazzo pants makes the figure look a tad bottom-heavy, plus the contrasting color of the tunic creates a strong horizontal line right across the middle of the figure. The only saving grace is that the silky fabric produces some pleasing vertical folds.

Camouflage Chic Rating: **C–**

RULE 4

WATCH YOUR BALANCE!

and perfectly proportioned—or tall or skinny and totally out of balance. Everybody's favorite plus-size model, Emme, for instance, may be a little chunky by some standards, but she still looks great in most clothing styles because her five-foot, eleven-inch body is well proportioned.

Proportion

I think I'm kind of weird looking. If I could change the way I look, I'd like to have longer legs, smaller feet, a smaller nose, and I'd even like, you know, bigger . . . But the one thing I wouldn't change is my hands. I think I've got very capable-looking hands.

—MEG RYAN, actress

Proportion is essentially the way various parts of your body relate spatially to the other parts—how long your legs are in relation to your torso, how wide your rib cage is in relation to your hips, how low or high your breasts are on your chest, etc. All this makes a big difference in how you look in various styles of clothing. Even a simple deviation in shoulder width can affect the way a garment hangs. Which is why something that looks terrific on your best friend, who wears the same size as you do, can look terrible on you—and vice versa.

Fashion is architecture; it is a matter of proportions.

—COCO CHANEL, designer

One of the most common reasons for looking fat in clothes is bad balance—that is, the proportions of your clothes are out of sync with the proportions of your body. *Bad balance reinforces figure flaws, while good balance de-emphasizes them.* Our mission, here in Rule 4, is to nudge everything into perfect balance.

Remember that proportions are *not* necessarily height or weight issues. You can be big or short

It's also why some women look better, or worse, in skirts, tube tops, or capri pants.

Balance Adjustments

To fine-tune *your* balance, we'll have to zero in on whatever specific proportions are throwing it off. But before we do that, let's start with the big picture and do a quick sweep of some **universal balance basics**—rules of thumb that help slim and trim no matter what shape you are.

Universal Balance Basics

• **Long over short or narrow and short over long or full.** This means a long top (jacket, cardigan, tunic, whatever) is best with a short skirt or narrow pants. And conversely, a cropped top is better with a longer skirt or fuller pants. Why? In part, because this proportion separates the body into thirds, rather than halves, which is more interesting and pleasing to the eye.

Since designers are always experimenting with new looks, they often bend this rule—always, mind you, on statuesque models. As a civilian, you want to think twice before breaking it. A snug cropped top and skinny pants (short over narrow) are a risky combo for most women. Ditto for a slouchy jacket over baggy pants or full skirt (long/full over full).

The bottom line: Exceptions to this basic balance rule can *sometimes* work.

The rule on the other hand, *always* works. The taller, thinner, and more evenly proportioned you are, the more you can get away with breaking this rule (and, for that matter, most of the others in this book).

• **Skim, don't cling.** Garments that skim and contour your body give you a nice slim look. Garments that cling to it make you look fatter. I can't stress this one enough. Tight clothing can make even a model look fat. (See Rule 5 for fit essentials.)

• **Skirts are most slimming when they fall close to your body and are longer than they are wide.** This makes for maximum elongation. You're in dangerous territory when a skirt is so short that it looks more square than rectangular. Although A-line skirts can help conceal bulges, they are style risks since they can come across as dull and matronly. Consider trumpet skirts instead.

• **Ultrawide shoulders, big collars, and wide-legged slacks** add unnecessary dimension and thus are potential fat-makers. (Please see Rule 11.)

• **Floor-length coats and winter skirts will make you look

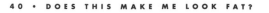

shorter. They tend to anchor you to the ground like a fire hydrant. The length is less risky in lightweight, fluid fabrics, but as a rule, ankle length is as long as anyone should ever go—except with evening gowns.

- **The wider the pant leg, the softer and more fluid the fabric should be—and the longer the length.** No wide, stiff palazzos. Narrow pants can be worn shorter. *Most* slacks are *most* slenderizing when they are straight and long.

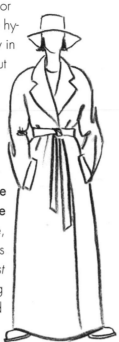

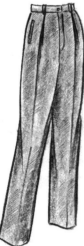

- **Pleated pants are slimming only when they are extremely well cut.** Pleats must lie flat, and the waistband must be easy fitting. Say no to trousers that are tight in the tummy, stretch tightly across the derriere, are ultrafull, have large or visible front or back pockets, or flirt with other excess detailing (see Rule 5).

- **Overgathering or excess pleating on any garment is fattening.**

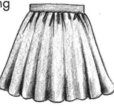

- **Shorter hair generally makes you look taller.** When the neck shows, the figure looks elongated. Anything bulky around the neck (hair included) will make you look shorter.

- **A tiny bit of shoulder padding** gives a lift, which makes the figure look longer.

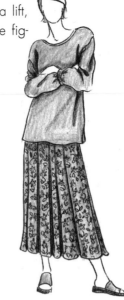

Your Specific Proportions

> *I have small sloping shoulders, so I do not wear huge shoulder pads. I'm not sure I want to put on eighties clothes again.*
>
> —Jane Seymour, **actress**

Now let's get to *you* specifically. Before we can talk about what styles will best balance your particular proportions, you obviously have to be very familiar with what your proportions are. So sit down for a minute—or better yet, stand naked in front of a full-length mirror—and give some serious thought to which parts of your body could use a little balancing. It shouldn't be too hard to figure out. Chances are you already know.

The biggest balance problems have to do with how the top half of your body relates to the bot-

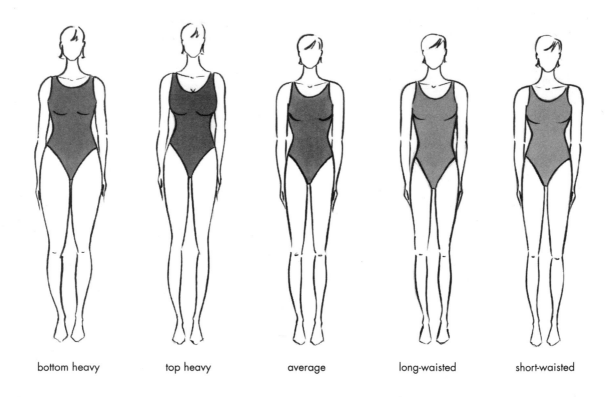

| bottom heavy | top heavy | average | long-waisted | short-waisted |

tom half. So here are your choices in the "major proportional discrepancy" category. Are you

1. bottom-heavy,
2. top-heavy,
3. long-waisted (long torso/short legs), or
4. short-waisted (short torso/long legs)?

What do you think? Are you one of the above, a combination of two, or none? If your answer is *none of the above,* you're probably fairly evenly proportioned, and you have my permission to skip the next couple of pages. But before you go, let me say a few words about the **short-waisted/long-waisted variation**—because while it's easy to tell if you're top-heavy or bottom-heavy, it's a wee bit trickier to pinpoint waist position. So here are a couple of easy ways to tell:

1. Feel around the bottom of your rib cage and see how close it is to your hipbone. If it's practi-

cally sitting right on top of it, you're short-waisted. If the distance is more than a hand span, say four inches or so, then you're long-waisted. Average is somewhere in between.

2. Turn up the heat, strip down, stand with your back to a full-length mirror, and look at your reflected backside with a compact or hand mirror. Notice if there is more expanse of skin between your waist and shoulders (which would make you long-waisted) or between your waist and the bottom of your buttocks (which would make you short-waisted). If your waist falls in the middle you're average.

3. And easiest of all, just think on this: If the proportion goddess suddenly appeared and offered you a few extra inches in the legs or the torso, where would you take them? If you'd like your bonus inches in the legs, chances are you're long-waisted. If you'd like them in the torso, you're probably short-waisted, and if you

don't care, you most likely have an average waist. There you go.

Now, if after this fun little bit of self-scrutiny you still believe you're relatively well proportioned, skip on ahead while the rest of us get balanced—which is going to be fairly easy since Rules 1, 2, and 3 have already given us an excellent start. **Dressing in dark neutral monochromes and going for vertical lines are terrific across-the-board equalizers**—something to always keep in mind. Okay—balance solutions for long waists and short waists.

If You're Short-Waisted . . .

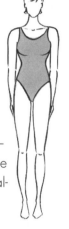

Because your torso is short, your legs are probably relatively long—that's the good news, since, as I've mentioned, *height is perceived according to leg length*. So the trick is to maintain the long-legged look—which will make you look taller and slimmer—while at the same time adding a little extra length to your torso for better balance. Here's how:

• **Create vertical and strong diagonal lines above the waist** with long shawl collars, deep V necks, shirts open to the waist (over camisoles, tank tops, T-shirts, or turtlenecks), long beads or chains (twenty-six inches or longer), and long scarves.

• **Add an inch or two with mandarin and stand-up collars.**

• With trousers, **wear tops (shells, vests, Ts, etc.) that fall an inch or so below your beltline.** With flat-front narrow pants and skirts, wear tops (*without* bottom binding) to top of hipbone.

• If you prefer to tuck in your blouses, make sure you **blouson them out and over the waistline.** And think about lowering or removing the belt loops on your slacks and wearing your belt *below* the waistband instead of on it. I do it all the time and it really works. It's a favorite in my personal camouflaging arsenal.

• **If you wear belts, keep them the same color as your top**—it adds an inch or two to the torso instantly. If you're relatively slim through the hips, you could even try a wide elastic belt worn very low on the waist—the bottom of the belt then reaches an inch or two below your natural waist. Then, when you blouse your top over the belt, it looks as if the bottom of the belt is on your actual waistline. I like this one a lot, too.

• **Wearing a narrow belt or chain on the hips will also lengthen the torso,** but if you're at all hippy, keep the belt the same color as the outfit and don't drop it too low—you don't want an obvious horizontal line across the widest part of your hips. Careful with this one! The cut and drape of the outfit have to be flawless.

- Slacks usually look terrific on long legs, **but don't lose your leg length** by wearing tops too long. In theory, the longer your top, the shorter the bottom looks.

AND FINALLY—SHORT-WAISTED? TRY PETITES!

This last tip is the one you might just love me for the most. All short-waisted women who have ever had problems with fit should at least try petite sizes for jackets, tops, and dresses. They may not work for you, but they are definitely worth a try. Petites are based not on weight or size, but on proportion—and that proportion is short-waisted. So don't be fooled by the word *petite*. It doesn't really mean small. There are even plus-size petites! A name change is long overdue, if you ask me.

I always knew I was short-waisted, but for some reason it took me forever to figure out that I should be wearing a petite top—and I'm in the business! At five feet, six inches, it just never occurred to me that I could be a petite. All I knew was that I could never find dresses or fitted jackets that looked right. I finally gave up on dresses altogether, and with jackets, I was just resigned to constantly rolling up sleeves and altering shoulders and hemlines. It was a drag, but hey, Calvin didn't make petites.

Even when we were getting my wardrobe together for my TV show (sixty-five outfits for sixty-five episodes) and had to have all the jackets and tops

altered, it still didn't occur to me that petite tops were the solution. In retrospect I feel pretty dumb for not figuring it out. But the amazing thing is that it never dawned on any of the other fashion pros who were working on the project either. They were so used to dealing with models that petite wasn't part of their fashion vocabulary either. Anyway, suffice it to say that when I inadvertently tried on my first petite jacket, it was as if I'd found God—a total revelation. Now I shop for jackets and dresses in the petite department (Emanuel Petites fit me like a dream), and slacks in the regular department.

I can't guarantee you'll get the fit satisfaction I did, but as I said, it's definitely worth a shot. Trying on is free. Try a few different sizes from a few different labels, since they're all proportioned slightly differently. If, like me, you're petite only on top, check out designers who cut their regular collections in petite sizes as well. That way you can easily match up your petite tops with regular bottoms.

Proportion is so important, as is how fabric curves around the form. When these elements serve the body, you get clothes that give women power. And power is sexy.

—ALBER ELBAZ, designer

If You're Long-Waisted . . .

Being long-waisted has advantages and disadvantages, too. Dresses, tops, jackets, and skirts are easier to fit. Plus, you have more room above the waist for interesting layering. **The main disadvantage is that you have proportionally short legs.** Generally, the longer your waist, the shorter your legs. So the goal is to visually lengthen the legs. Here's how to do it:

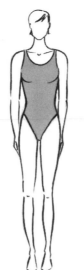

- **Skirts are safer than pants** because the eye doesn't discern where the leg begins as readily. Best lines: Long, slim skirts usually make you look taller. Shortish skirts are fine if your legs are good, but no micro-minis. Because there is relatively little leg to cover, the skirt ends up looking like a little square piece of material, instead of a rectangle—and legs look even shorter.

- **Worst pant cuts:** Pedal pushers, capris, ultra-tapered styles, and any pants even vaguely resembling hip-huggers. Even low-riding jeans will totally throw your proportions out of whack. The lower pants ride on your hips, the shorter your legs will look and the more abnormally long your torso will appear.

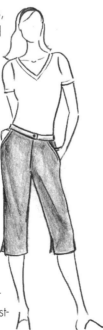

- **Best pant cuts:** Any high-waisted pants, especially classic trousers with great drape, straight, fairly narrow legs, and pleats that fall in lovely, elongating vertical lines. The higher waist-band will visually raise your waist a couple of inches, thus making your legs look longer. *No cuffs*—they'll shorten the leg. Always wear trousers with some of sort of heel, and let the pant leg fall over the shoe.

- Try **reverse layering** on top: Keep the outside layer shorter than the ones under it. Example: Start out with a simple dark monotone top and bottom—a longish top worn out over the narrow bottom. Then wear a shorter vest or slightly fuller, shorter pullover (about an inch or two shorter than your waist) over the base outfit. If it's a *slightly* different tone, color, or texture, the eye will register the higher division line and your waist will look higher, your legs longer.

- Wide belts can help raise the waist and lengthen legs **if the belt is in the same color as your bottom,** *not* your top.

- **Slightly Empire-waisted dresses** are technically a perfect balance—just be careful that the designs aren't too cute and girly.

- Finally, there is one particular **evening silhouette** that I find particularly unflattering to long-waisted women: A long dress or gown that hugs the body like a glove, then flares out below the knee. Even when worn with high heels, it accentuates the shortness of the legs. First, because it hugs the body, it clearly defines the long torso, then the flare in the skirt breaks the line of the leg in two, emphasizing the shortness of both the thighs and the lower legs.

I've seen two very long waisted actresses (Claire Danes and Courtney Cox) in this particular style, and even though both women are lovely and the dresses were tasteful, the proportion did them in, and they ended up looking a little stunted. They've both looked 100 percent better in other gowns. Best ideas: styles that fall straight from below the bust or long tapered columns.

If You Are Bottom-Heavy . . .

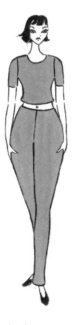

Your shoulders and rib cage are quite a bit narrower than your hips and thighs—even at your fighting weight. Any extra weight settles below your waist, in the hips, thighs, derriere, and sometimes on the legs. Your bust is usually average to small, face and neck generally slender.

Sound familiar? If it doesn't describe you, it probably does one of your close friends. It's one of the most common balance discrepancies going. There are basically three rebalance remedies: 1. Add some extra dimension to the top; 2. reduce dimension on the bottom; or 3. redirect attention from the broadness below to the slimness above. Here's how you do it:

• **Always wear shoulder pads** (but watch the size!). Shoulder pads are the best way to add a little extra dimension up top, so don't worry whether *Vogue* says they're in or out. They are fabulous equalizers in any season. As they extend and broaden the shoulder, they allow your top to hang in a straighter line from the shoulder to the hip, producing a more balanced, slimming silhouette.

In order for shoulder pads to work their magic, though, they must be the right size and shape. Too broad or thick (think Joan Collins in *Dynasty*), and you can lose your neck and end up looking like a Notre Dame fullback; too small and thin, and they're ineffectual. So go to the most comprehensive notions store in your area and experiment until you find ones that give you a pleasing natural balance. You'll find that some shapes seem to be better suited to specific types of garments. The pads with rounder, softer edges generally work better with knits and unstructured softer garments. The squarer-edged shapes are a natural with tailored styles and garments with a sharp seam at the shoulder. It's a good idea to have both styles in your closet.

If your tops and blouses already have shoulder pads sewn in, check to make sure they're the right size for you. If not, snip them out and simply wear the garment over your store-bought pads.

Also, remember that you can take trickier garments such as coats and jackets to a tailor for a **shoulder pad makeover**—they can be enlarged or reduced for a very nominal fee. There might be some life left in those old eighties jackets yet.

On the subject of jackets: Since a lot of them come prepadded in the shoulders, watch out that you don't double pad. If the jacket has shoulder pads, reduce or eliminate the pad in your blouse. To paraphrase Dan Quayle, *The neck is a terrible thing to lose.*

Alert! Check that shoulder pads aren't visible under thin, white, or light-colored garments (should you ignore Rule 2 and wear them). It can bring your whole look down a peg. If they do show, think about wearing a slip, a camisole, or even a T-shirt over them. Plain white men's T-shirts (they come in small to X-large) can be cut and shaped to fit under or over just about anything—sleeves can be trimmed or eliminated, necklines can be scooped out, lengths adjusted. Just keep trimming with scissors until they fit the purpose.

No stitching, hemming, or skills needed. It's not terribly chic, but hey, it does the trick!

- Before we leave the subject of padding: **If you're wide-hipped and very small busted, you could consider a padded bra** to help the balance in certain outfits. I'm not talking fifties retro va-va-voom here, just a little more equilibrium. There are some beautiful, wonderfully designed, contoured, and slightly padded seamless bras on the market. They add just a hint of extra natural dimension—and sometimes that's all it takes for a garment to hang a little better. (Check Playtex's Thank Goodness It Fits line and Victoria's Secret Perfect Silhouette bra, among others.) Or you could even try Curves, those soft silicone inserts that slip into your bra and are supposed to look amazingly natural under clothes. I haven't tried them myself, but they are apparently the no-muss, no-fuss version of dreaded implants. Think of them as *explants*—harmless, painless, trouble-free. They even hug well—so they say. (Call 800-5-CURVES for more info.)

MAYBE YOU CAN USE THIS

While we're cutting up T-shirts, here's a bonus tip that's really going to sound odd, but I swear it works. Cut the sleeves out of T-shirts—along with a little bit of the body of the shirt—and wear them as perspiration shields under silk blouses and sleeveless shells—under jackets, of course. (They're easy enough to slip out of if you have to take off the jacket, which I rarely do.) Just slide them up the arm and them tuck them under your bra straps on top and the top of the bra on the sides (under the arm). They're great for stressful situations. Really saves the silk and cuts down on cleaning bills—for both the tops and the jackets.

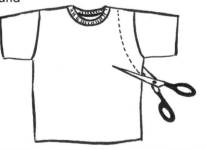

Also try:

- **Tailored and semitailored tops and jackets.** You need the extra shoulder width that set-in sleeves provide. No wimpy, round-shouldered sweater sets, and no dolman or raglan sleeves.

- **Layering.** Soft vests—hip length or longer—worn open, over a blouse or sweater, help pull together the top and bottom without looking boxy.

- **Scarves and shawls worn around the shoulders.** They add some dimension to the top for balance, as well as direct the eye up to the face and away from the broad bottom.

- **Boat necks, slightly wider lapels,** and even a subtle horizontal trim across the top. Just a hint of horizontal on top will help balance.

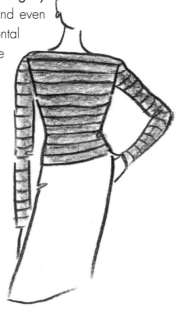

- **Tops that are somewhat loose**—at least not clingy. No tight bodysuits into full trousers—unless worn with a vest, cardigan, or jacket.

- **Waistlines and belts that are loose enough to be totally comfortable.** The more you cinch in your waist, the bigger your hips will look. If you do wear belts, keep them on the narrow side.

- **Soft, flowing skirts** that are cut slim and close to the body and that fall smoothly over hips without clinging. The natural drape forms elongating vertical lines. For a more tailored look, go for a tapered straight skirt or a gored trumpet style. Forget any kind of gathered skirts. They just add more width to the bottom of the figure, which you don't need.

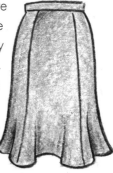

- **Well-tailored, well-cut basic trousers** with soft deep pleats that lie flat and fall in slimming vertical lines. The pants should just skim the body. Pant legs should fall straight from the hips and taper *slightly* at the ankles. Essentially pleated pants work only if they are flawlessly designed and drape like a dream. If there is any pull at the pleats, they'll make you look hippier. So beware of inexpensive pleated pants that have short, skimpy pleats that pouf out over the stomach. Also pass on slacks that are too wide, have ultra-full triple pleats or large front or back pockets, or flirt with other excess detailing. **It's always better**

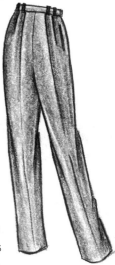

to invest in one really good pair of slacks that fit perfectly than in three pairs that don't quite cut the mustard.

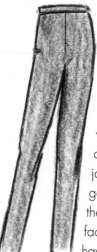

•Narrow, flat-front, side-zipper, pocketless pants. These can work, but it depends on the size of your thighs. If they're very big, you're generally better off in skirts or trousers. It also depends on what you pair them with. Flat-front pants could look great with a sweater or jacket, but *not* with a snug top. In general, they minimize bulk, but if they're the least bit tight, they can, in fact, highlight extra ounces unless they have some Lycra in them, in which case they can hold you in and be quite slimming (the slight stretch also makes them more comfortable). To cover the tummy, try tops that fall straight from the shoulder to the hipbone or below, without binding at the bottom. Straight-legged pants without Lycra need to be roomier through the hips and thighs.

• Side pockets. Depending on the cut and fabric, pants pockets can add an extra quarter inch or so to the hips—remember, more material equals extra inches. **Consider getting side pockets removed** and have the seam sewn up (unless you're like me and love the practicality of pockets). It's an easy alteration for even a semi-competent tailor. In the case of the pear-shaped body (*not* an Agatha Christie mystery), you'll also want to balance the top and bottom with shoulder pads and jacket cuts.

If You Are Top-Heavy . . .

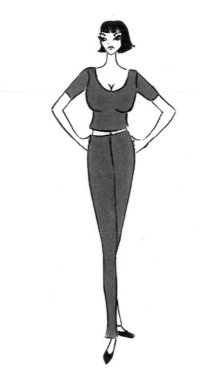

Your shoulders are wider than your hips. You tend to gain weight in the stomach, waist, bust, and maybe even through the upper back. Your waist is usually undefined, your hips are relatively slim, your derriere flat.

Broad shoulders, in and of themselves, are a fashion plus. They give clothes a nice solid base from which to drape and hang—just like a good solid wood hanger. But when broad shoulders are combined with a big bosom and/or large rib cage, belly, or back, you can end up looking hefty.

The best rebalance remedy here is to slim down the top as much as possible and to subtlely direct attention to your slimmest parts—either your great legs, narrow hips, or face. Theoretically, you could also achieve balance by adding a little bit more dimension to the bottom part of your body. But what's the point? You'll just end up looking big all over. Two big parts, after all, always equal a big whole—Fashion Math 101. So with that in mind, try the following ideas:

- First and foremost, **remove all shoulder pads.** If they're needed to help shape a garment, make sure they are the slimmest ones possible. And while the scissors are out, operate on any jackets or tops with epaulets on them. All epaulets have to go!

- **Wear unstructured styles and soft, fluid designs.** Light to midweight knits that just skim the body are a natural. Stay away from boxy, structured, blazer-type jackets—double-breasted jackets are especially deadly.

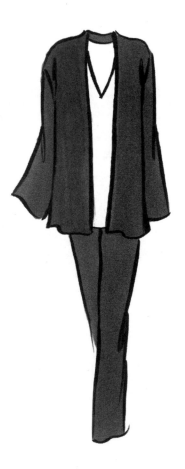

- **Avoid excess detailing on tops.** No patch pockets, dreaded epaulets, embroidery, wide collars, ruffles, large closures, etc. Simple tops, and blouses with plackets that hide buttons, are ideal (see Rule 12).

- **Think vertical above the waist**—V necks, shawl collars, and open necklines. No square necks, boat necks, or halters.

- **Keep pants on the narrow side.** Even classic trousers should be reasonably narrow-legged—and make sure the fabric is top quality so that it drapes well.

- **Try slim tunics over skinny pants,** tights, or narrow skirts. No bulky sweaters.

- **The right bra is essential.** You need ones that support and minimize (see Rule 8).

- **No wide belts** or short cropped tops.

> *In the gym, I see all kinds of women, all shapes and sizes. It's the models who are the anomalies.*
>
> —THANDIE NEWTON, actress

Minor Balance Discrepancies

The following variables are *not* a big deal—**definitely not worth even a minor obsession**—but they require some attention when slim is the goal. So . . . a few tips:

SHORT NECKS

The goal here is elongation.

- **Think vertical and diagonal necklines** (see Rule 3). Go for V necks, open collars. Don't cut off the neck abruptly with crew necks, boat necks, or blouses buttoned all the way up

- Don't bunch anything up around the neck—no complicated, closed-up collars, no ascots, bulky scarves, or thick turtlenecks. Try mid- to light-weight shallow mock turtles if you need more winter neck cover.

- Keep hair relatively short and off the neck.

- Avoid chokers, short necklaces, and other jewelry that focuses attention on the neck—such as long dangling earrings.

> *The key to a great silhouette is to keep the cut simple, the shape tenderly caressing, and the fabric rich.*
>
> —RALPH LAUREN, designer

LONG NECKS

Long necks are not a problem since they elongate the body. So if you have one, rejoice and take advantage of it. Turn collars up, wear turtlenecks or cowlnecks or both together. Try mandarin collars, scarves, and cuff necklaces. High boat necks that can shorten average necks are ideal for you. Also remember that a long beautiful swanlike neck can make quite a smashing statement when totally exposed and unadorned. So don't think you always have to cover it. For evening consider going for high drama by accentuating the neck by leaving shoulders and neck bare. Short hair, or upswept do's worn off the neck, would further accentuate your neck's grace.

HEAVY LEGS—CALVES AND ANKLES

Essentially everything you wear should be designed to focus attention elsewhere, which means:

- No tight or cropped pants, miniskirts, strappy shoes, or Manolo stilettos. The latter would be too delicate and make your leg look heavier in contrast.

- Match tones of hemline, hose, and shoes when possible. Shoes can be darker than hemline but never lighter. Hose can be lighter than shoes but never darker (never white, please!). The less contrast, the better.

- Best bets: Classic slacks, long fluid skirts, and sensible hemlines that fall at the narrowest part of the leg (see Rule 5).

- A well-fitted slim boot is a great look in winter.

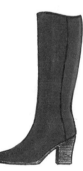

> *Darling, the legs aren't so beautiful. I just know what to do with them.*
>
> —MARLENE DIETRICH, actress

HEAVY ARMS AND BAT WINGS

Long sleeves are, of course, the number one answer for heavy arms. But the shape of the sleeve makes a big difference—not only in how well it camouflages but also in how slim you look in general. There are three key details to note: the size of the armhole, the fullness of the sleeve, and the length of the sleeve.

- Basically, a **higher armhole** makes you look thinner because it allows a nice long vertical silhouette from armpit to hip, which lengthens the torso and elongates the body. That's why we all looked so skinny in those snug seventies jackets. On the other hand, fuller arms need a fuller armhole and sleeve. So **look for sleeves that give you just enough ease around the upper arm for comfort, but not an inch more.** If sleeves are too full or too short, you'll look bigger all over.

- Make sure **sleeves taper at the wrist.** If they don't, get them altered. A slim wrist will make the whole arm look slimmer. Casually pushing up sleeves also gives that nice tapering effect.

- Whatever you do, **never wear tight sleeves of any kind!** Especially beware of those little short cap sleeves that cut into the upper arm. They're lethal on heavy upper arms! In fact, they're not great on anyone but a total twig. If you must go for short sleeves, make sure they fall straight from the shoulder, have a fairly wide opening, and are long enough to totally cover the bat wing—with nothing peeking out.

- If you want to go totally sleeveless, think **about draping a fabulous chiffon scarf or shawl over your shoulders**—a great look in the summer and still cool. Even though you can technically see through chiffon, nobody really looks. But scarf or no, watch the cut of the armhole. An abrupt arm-hole focuses attention on the upper arm—which is, needless to say, something you want to avoid.

BIG BELLIES

Stay away from belts and anything bulky around the waist. Big tops that cover but don't cling to the belly are naturals. Skirts are usually an easier fit than pants. Elasticized pants will work, but please cover up the elastic part.

And a Final Balance Tip for Everybody: Watch Your Tunic and Jacket Lengths!

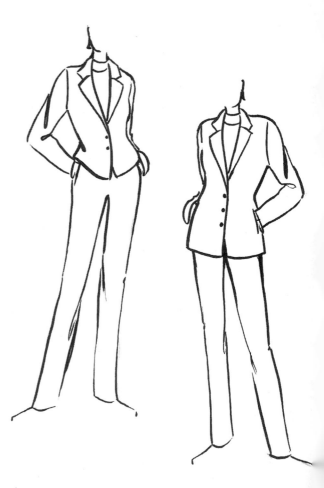

This is a little proportion thing that can turn into a big balance problem without your even noticing it. And because it's so subtle even your best friend might not notice. But what you both will undoubtedly recognize is that something seems off and that you look a little chubbier than usual. That's because tops that are too short or long can make you look considerably shorter and/or heavier.

Many women fall into the too-long trap because they're very conscious of covering up full thighs and rears. So they'll wear a nice long jacket or a long, full overblouse or sweater. Basically, it's a sound idea. But often the tops are so long that they cut into the length of the leg and end up shortening the whole body, which in turn makes the woman stockier. So remember, **your top should be long enough only to fully cover the problem area, not an inch longer.**

Theoretically, then, short tops should make you look taller, which they generally do—if you're slim-hipped. That's why those little cropped tops look so cute on skinny teenagers. But if you carry any extra weight below the waist, as the majority of women do, you have to be careful. If tops are too short, they can emphasize big hips and derrieres. So the length of your tops and jackets has to be perfect— long enough to cover problem areas and short enough to give you leg length.

Exception: If you have a **prominent rear end** and wear skirts, you can often wear jackets that hang straight and end just at the top of the buttocks. If the jacket is well tailored, you'll get a nice straight line in the back and your rear will be less noticeable. This concept also works with well-cut trousers. Please forget about skinny pants altogether. They are not for you.

There's one other factor to toss into the balance mix, besides, of course, your particular body shape, and that is the shape and color of both the top and bottom of the outfit. The general rule of thumb here: **The more color contrast between top and bottom, the more crucial the length of the top.** The closer they are in color, the less exact you have to be, because the eye will perceive the top and bottom as a whole unified silhouette. It won't immediately discern the dividing line between top and bottom.

> *I can't think of any woman that I know who looks in the mirror and thinks, I'm hot.*
>
> —JEANNE TRIPPLEHORN, actress

IF IT DOESN'T FIT, GET RID OF IT!

contains only clothes that fit! (See page 127 for closet organization tips.)

Here's the deal with fit: Clothes that are *too big* can make you look fat, and clothes that are *too small* can make you look fat, and clothes that *are tight* will *definitely* make you look fat—with the exception of a Hervé Leger–type dress, which, while tight, has enough heavy-duty Lycra in it to choke an elephant.

Elasticized dresses aside, remember that our mantra is always **skim, don't cling.** You've heard it before; you'll hear it again. It's crucial. You will always look your slimmest in clothes that fit perfectly. Note that size is not synonymous with fit. All manufacturers' sizes vary since they all use different fit models for sizing. (I, for instance, am a size four in Ellen Tracy pants and a ten in Richard Tyler!) So look at the garments themselves, not the size labels.

> *If you wear clothes a teeny bit too small you immediately gain ten pounds.*
>
> —MARCIA GAY HARDEN, actress

We all have garments hanging in our closets that fit just badly enough to make us look fat every time we put them on. So what are they doing in there? Are we into sartorial masochism?

Do yourself a favor and **get everything that doesn't fit** *out* of your closet. When something fits well, it can make you look five pounds thinner and ten times better. When it fits badly, it can turn your Armani into Army-Navy and plump you up like a double down pillow. A good closet is a closet that

> *My clothes cannot be too short or too tight or something I'm going to be worrying about. There's no time.*
>
> —GERALDINE FERRARO, politician

What Is Good Fit?

In a nutshell, a garment that fits well is neither too skimpy nor too bulky and is in no way constricting.

It falls gracefully and hits your body where it is designed to—not above or below the area. There are no extraneous bumps, lumps, creases, puckers, pulls, gaps, droops, bags, etc. Key areas to watch are shoulders, bust, waist, derriere, crotch, arms, and legs.

The following is a list of common fit offenses that are guaranteed to add extra ounces (or pounds) just where you don't want them. Steer clear of all garments possessing any of these features. If you already own some, get them altered or replace them.

> Comfort is everything. Why go out for an evening and be miserable. . . . I'm not going to be squishing and pinching and pushing and pulling. Oh no!
>
> —PHYLICIA RASHAD, actress

Fit Problems That Add Pounds

TOO SMALL

- **Tight waistbands.** Tight waistbands are one of the top fat-makers. We all have flesh on our bones. We're supposed to. That's how we earthlings are built. But when that flesh is compressed or squeezed, it pops out somewhere else, and bingo, you look fat. That's what happens with tight waists if you have even one little extra ounce in the vicinity. As the waist gets squeezed, little (or maybe big) bulges are created under the rib cage (just above the tight waistband) and on the top of the hip (right below the waistband). It happens with skirts, pants, shorts, tights, even panty hose.

A loose waistband, on the other hand, doesn't squeeze anything. It just skims the waist and allows the garment to fall gracefully. **If you can't slip a couple of fingers between yourself and the waistband, it's probably too tight.** You will actually *feel slimmer* when the waist fits properly. It makes all the difference in the world—even in hang-out garments like sweatpants. In fact, in some cases you can do a quick sweatpant fix yourself by simply yanking out the old tight elastic and replacing it with a bigger piece. All you do is make a little slit near the seam on the inside of the waistband, reach through the slit with tweezers, grab hold of the old elastic, snip it, and pull it out. Put a new bigger piece in by attaching it to a safety pin and sliding it into the hole and around the waistband. Either sew the ends together or tie them off.

- **Sausage-encased arms.** If your arms are a little heavy, don't wear long sleeves so tight that they make your arms look like sausages. This warning applies to vegetarians and nonvegetarians alike.

- **Smiling crotches** are not happy crotches. They are those dreaded horizontal lines that you get across the front of your pants, near the crotch, when the pants are one or two sizes too small. Pants that are tight through the crotch also tend to be tight across the thighs and emphasize lower hip bulge (a.k.a. saddlebags) if it's there. So if your crotch is smiling, smile back and then eighty-six the pants. Tight pants are also unflattering if you have a belly bulge, unless the pants have enough heavy-duty Lycra in them to help hold you in. (*Possible* exception: classic jeans. When they fit perfectly, they can also hold you in a bit.)

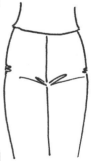

- **Pulled pleats and/or gaping pockets** add instantaneous pounds. Trouser and skirt pleats should always lie flat so that you get the benefit of the vertical lines. As soon as they pouf out, so do you. Words of wisdom from custom designer Rob Kinch:

> Large women come in and say, "Don't give me any pleats on slacks because they make me look fat." The first thing I say is, "No, *no* pleats make you look fat. Let me make the pleat on you." A pleat is the best thing for a wide-hipped woman, providing that the pleat is in the right place, stays closed, and has a perfect vertical line. Once you have that vertical line running right down the center of your leg you look really slender.

- **Seam pulls or puckers anywhere on your body.** A seam that pulls or puckers gives the impression that there is something big underneath making it happen. And there might be.

- **Zipper placket gaping—stressed zippers.** Same as above.

- **Pants that cut up between the buttocks** (usually because of a rise that is too high) **or stretch tightly across the derriere or thighs.** Tight jeans are a common culprit in this category.

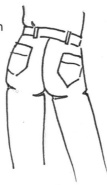

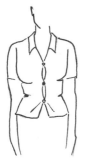

•**Gaping buttons and other closures.** A top that pulls at its closures and allows sneak peeks at the bra underneath is fattening—whether you're skinny, fat, small-busted, or large-busted. If this happens on any of your tops, either sew on a tiny hook and eye or small pieces of Velcro or simply sew the darn thing closed permanently and slip the blouse over your head.

- **Clingy knits.** Knits that *skim* the body are fine. It's just when they cling that they're deadly, since they then outline absolutely any and every imperfection. Sometimes, though, they can look good *under* a second layer. So try them under vests, dusters, and other loose-fitting tops.

•**Tight, stretchy tops.** Stretchy tops can be great, but they can also be dangerous if the fabric is not heavy enough. When most of us sit down and lean over a tad, a little roll of flesh mysteriously appears between the bust and the waistline—even on relatively skinny women (a belly roll!). Well, that little roll shows in thin, tight, stretchy tops. This never would have occurred to me had I not inadvertently looked down at some notes in my lap while I was interviewing Cheryl Tiegs on my show. Lo and behold, there was this little roll above my belt—and I was at my fighting weight, too! Cheryl, being the kind soul that she is, assured me during the break that it was hardly noticeable, but of course it totally ruined my concentration for the rest of the show. Needless to say, I never wore that top—or any other lightweight, stretchy top—again. Watch that you don't suffer the same indignity!

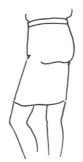

- **Skirts that curve in under buttocks.** Skirts look slimmest when they fall straight over the derriere. When they start curving under, you're in trouble.

- **Bias-cut skirts and dresses.** I totally love bias skirts. They're slinky without being overly clingy and move with a kind of magical grace—think Carolyn Bessette Kennedy's wedding dress. Unfortunately, they're rather unforgiving when it comes to tummy bulges, large derrieres, or saddle-bags. So, should you possess any of those features, either wear a top that covers, try ultra-control-top panty hose or shapewear (see Rule 8), or give bias-cut skirts a miss altogether. And always check your full-body profile and rear view in a full-length mirror.

- **Derriere hanging out under jacket or tunic.** Regulation-length jackets should reach down to the bottom of your buttocks. You don't want half moons showing below your jacket hem in the back. You might not see yourself from the back, but other people do.

> *I don't wear things that are tight on my hips. I like to wear dresses and show leg and have a free-flowing line.*
>
> —LELA ROCHON, **actress**

TOO BIG

- **Droopy T-shirt necklines.** This is something you see a lot because a lot of us like to wear *overlarge* T-shirts—which, not surprisingly, come with *overlarge* necklines. 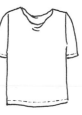 Thing is, it usually makes your neck look fat. I happened to catch Rosie the other day, and there she was in a V-neck sweater and a droopy-necked T-shirt. Since I generally admire her fashion choices, I wanted to call her immediately and say, "Hey Rosie, it's Leah, pull that neckline back up."

- **Oversized "boyfriend" jackets.** They're a bit démodé at the moment, but oversize jackets can still look quite good on *tall, thin women*. 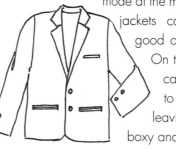 On the other hand, they can overwhelm small to average women, leaving them looking boxy and stocky.

- **Extra jacket fabric above the waist.** This often occurs when short-waisted women wear fitted jackets. Try petite sizes and have the jackets you already own altered.

TRICK

If a T-shirt neck is too big, try wearing the T-shirt backward—it's usually a much more flattering line. I do this so much it's practically a signature look, which I suppose is a little pathetic, since I would rather Armani be my signature look, but there it is. Even if you think the neck fits, try it backward to see how the line looks on you.

- **Badly hanging hems.** Because of tummies, rears, swaybacks, and various other figure challenges, hems often don't fall straight. They should. Have them measured and altered by a professional.

- **Big armholes.** If your arms are more or less normal size, you don't need big armholes (a.k.a. armscyes) in shirts, dresses, and jackets. They can, in fact, make you look much bigger than you are. The reason everybody looked so skinny in the seventies, besides the fact that some of us actually were, was that most clothing was designed with very high, narrow armholes. In general, the higher the armhole, the slimmer you'll look. Don't sacrifice comfort, though, and always consider what you'll be wearing under the garment. (Exceptions: kimono sleeves and sleeveless tanks and tops.)

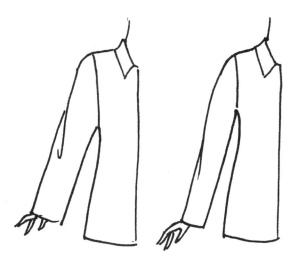

- **Ultrawide sleeves.** Slimmer sleeves usually make you look slimmer all over. If sleeves are too wide, they can broaden you as well. The best sleeve gives you enough room to maneuver about without extra bulk and has a slight taper from the armhole to the wrist. "You're always going to look a little more slender if you can see air and dead space between your arm and your body," says our custom designer friend Rob Kinch. "Most of the time sleeves are so big that it's just one big mass of fabric, which is not so pretty."

- **Sliding shoulder pads.** Nothing looks quite as silly as a shoulder pad in the middle of your back. While it won't exactly make you look fat, you will look slightly deformed, which is no more desirable. Make sure that shoulder pads are attached with Velcro or thread, affixed to bra straps, or otherwise well set.

- **Extra-long sleeves.** Long sleeves should hit just about at your wrist bone. And shirtsleeves shouldn't hang more than a half inch or so below jacket sleeves. If you find that your sleeves are always too long, you might be in the wrong size. You might want to try petites. I was forever rolling up my sleeves before my petite revelation. *One little exception:* If you're full through the hips, it's best to avoid long sleeves that fall *exactly* at the jacket hem, since they reinforce the horizontal line. In that case, hem your sleeves just a little above or below the wrists.

- **Overextended shoulders.** If your shoulder pads extend too far beyond your natural shoulder line, you'll look wider.

- **Falling shoulder seams.** Set-in sleeve seams should sit at, or just a wee bit outside, the shoulder bone, not inside.

- **Droopy crotch.** There's nothing like a droopy crotch to make your legs look shorter. And when

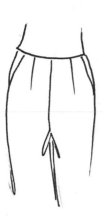

your legs look shorter, you know what happens—FAT! If you're in a skinny phase at the moment, there's a good chance that some of your pants are too big for you. Check them out. If the waist is ultraloose, the crotch will droop. Either get the pants altered or store them away in a box marked "Fat Clothes" until your weight swings back around, or try the following little trick. But whatever you do, just don't let 'em droop.

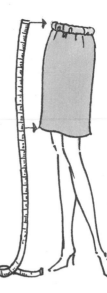

Hemlines

Hemlines depend on only three things: your body, the style of the garment, and the shoes you wear. They do not depend on what's in this season, because that will change next season and, as we know, it's basically all hype anyway. A few sea-

---

TRICK

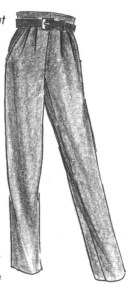

This is one of my all-time favorites. It works best with *wonderfully well-cut pleated drapy slacks* (the ones I do it with are lightweight gabardine and supersoft suede).

When slacks are too large—the waist feels too loose and the crotch is too low—pull them up till the crotch is where it should be and the waistline is an inch or more *above* your natural waist. Then tuck in your top and wear an inch-wide belt *below* the waistband. The high waist makes your legs look a lot longer (all of a sudden you're two inches taller). Plus, the drape seems to hide any tummy bulge and instantly slims you down. Amazingly enough, this works whether you are long- or short-waisted or even a little hippy. It might *not* work if you're too heavy, but it's worth a try. The key, though, is the cut of the pants—they must have a great drape to them. Try it. If it works, go for broke and remove the belt loops.

> *When it comes to length, I say freedom of choice.*
>
> —KARL LAGERFELD, designer

sons back Marc Jacobs had a big hit with his six-hundred-dollar-plus below-the-knee retro-schoolgirl pleated skirt. The fashion press called it "flirty and purty," and maybe it was on Shalom and Kate and 3.2 percent of the other Gen Xers, but honestly it was a disaster for the average gal on the street. Although Marc thoughtfully sewed the accordion pleats down to the hip, the skirt was still *purty dowdy* on all but the world's slimmest hips—and a very awkward length for all nonmodels. If I remember, Shalom wore hers with supertrashy Manolos and a sexy, tight, see-through top—for that modern-couture juxtaposition of sensibilities that works *only* on catwalks.

Then for fall 1998 they were showing these awful to-the-floor lengths that had everybody looking as if they were nailed to the ground and were a pain to walk in. So enjoy length trends vicariously, but do what design genius Giorgio Armani suggests in real life—"find your ideal lengths and don't veer too far away from them."

WHAT IS YOUR IDEAL HEM LENGTH?

> *I look great in a miniskirt. It's all how you think about life.*
>
> —IVANA TRUMP, socialite/entrepreneur

Skirts: Since there are no hemline rules in fashion anymore, everybody's entitled to their own opinion on length. **But the bottom line is this: If you have great legs, show them; if you don't, don't.** Tina Turner can wear her skirts as short as she wants to. Hillary Clinton cannot. That's rule number one.

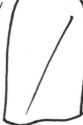

Rule number two has to do with common sense and propriety. The more conservative your environment is, the more conservative your hemline should be—unless, of course, you're out to rock the boat.

After that, it's a matter of the style and cut of a particular outfit and the shoes you'll be wearing with it. **In general, straight, narrow skirts look better on the short side—at least just above the knee. Fuller, more fluid skirts look more graceful if they are longer.** But to really zero in on your perfect *individual* hem lengths, you need to do a little experimentation to see which lengths best flatter your legs.

Experiment: Gather together a tape measure, a few pairs of shoes with different heel heights, a large scarf (or sarong, fabric piece, or even a long elastic-waisted skirt or slip), and a friend (any little helper over six years old will do; this experiment is exempt from child labor laws). A patient tailor is a good second choice if your friends or children are busy. Stand in front of a full-length mirror. Put on a pair of shoes and wrap the fabric (or whatever) around your body like a skirt with the "hem" just above the floor. Then slowly roll it at the waist, watching it very carefully until it hits a spot where your leg looks good. Stop there and have your friend measure the distance from the waist to the hemline. That measurement marks the longest you should wear skirts. Write down the measurement. Repeat the procedure to determine your best short length. Write that down too. Now go to your closet and try on a few skirts. Are they just right, or do they need to be lengthened or shortened? Remember that even half an inch can make a difference. If a straight skirt needs shortening, check to see if it also needs to be tapered to maintain its proportions. Before you actually hem anything, though, make sure to pin each garment to your new measurements just to be sure. The length may be right for your legs, but it has to be right for the proportions of the outfit, too.

I like for a skirt to fall one or two inches below the fingertips.

—MARCIA GAY HARDEN, actress, on *her* perfect length

A few tips and thoughts to consider as you're experimenting:

• Rob Kinch feels that short skirts are usually most flattering when they fall right around a certain part of the knee. "There's a little part of a woman's leg that goes in at the knee on the inside—a little indentation," he explains. "If you finish the skirt above that indentation, you'll be surprised how long and lean your leg will look. Many women will go right *below* that indentation so that you see the *widest* part of their knee, which makes them look very large and their knees not very pretty." Definitely something to check out!

• **A hemline that hits at the heaviest part of your leg adds pounds.** So if your legs are skinny, you can wear your longer skirts around midcalf—which is the heaviest part of the lower leg. If you have heavy legs, long skirts would look better

hemmed lower, at the narrowest part of the calf. As you experiment, see if this holds true for you.

• Since you always want to get vertical lines from a skirt, **it should be longer than it is wide.** Which is why fuller skirts usually look better a little longer and straight skirts a little shorter.

• Wearing a skirt longer than midcalf can make you look matronly—especially if you're short. **This length requires a triple check** and is another thing to look for as you experiment. Just above the ankle can be a graceful length, but is not recommended for women with thick ankles. As for ultralong skirts that fall below the ankle—well, that's an extremely tough length to make work with anything but evening gowns. Frankly, I wouldn't suggest it.

• **Skirts with side slits** are a natural if you have good legs. Skirts with *front* slits, on the other hand, never move very gracefully and are pretty unflattering on everybody.

If I have to adjust my clothes and worry about anything hanging out when I sit down it drives me crazy. So short skirts are out.

—GLORIA ESTEFAN, singer

Pant hems: Pant hems change from season to season just like skirt hems. One season long bell-bottoms are de rigueur, the next season clam diggers, pedal pushers, and capris are all the rage. What's a girl to do? Same as always—**figure what's right for you and stick to it!**

A few tips:

- Short, skinny pants are *not* good on heavy or short legs.

- Wide pants worn with flat shoes look best hemmed on the short side—that is, they should not fall over the shoe. If you're in the least bit heavy, you should probably have wide pants tapered in *a bit*—not too much. You might need the width through the thighs, but do you really need the same width around the calves? Probably not. Pants that are too wide will make you look square and boxy. **A little gradual taper from, say, mid-thigh down elongates the figure.**

- Soft, fluid, silky wide pants can be worn with heels (especially for evening) but should be longer and tapered so that the pants break a tiny bit, puddle around the ankle, and fall just a wee bit over the shoe. If the pants are not tapered and do fall over the shoe, you can trip and find yourself facedown on the carpet—never a good look.

One last word—**most good stores do alterations.** Banana Republic, J. Crew, and Club Monaco, for instance, now offer basic tailoring—hems and a little nip or taper—for *free* on nonsale items. If you're spending a considerable amount of money, most other retailers should do it for free as well. Should they resist, try the old "It's free for men, why not for women?" ploy. If you plan to wear heels with the pants, make sure you either have some with you or that the store provides you with a pair. (See Chapter 4 for more alteration tips.)

RULE 6

RUN FOR COVER!

muumuu is not what I would call subtle or stylish—except perhaps on the most distant of South Sea islands. Ditto for caftans, burnooses, and chadors—except in the Middle East. When in those distant regions, of course, feel free to indulge in indigenous dress. It's very tasteful to be sensitive to, and respectful of, regional diversity. Back in our neck of the woods, however, the sort of cover-ups you want to think about are **shawls and scarves, cleverly layered pieces, jackets, vests, cardigans (worn or wrapped), and sarongs for summer and beach.**

Larger women, I find, follow the old tent theory—if it's big enough and they hide under it, they think no one will know what's underneath. But the only thing wrong with a tent is everybody does know what's underneath—they figure that's why you wore it.

—ROB KINCH, **custom designer**

I may weigh more than most people, but why not flatter my shape instead of covering it up?

—EMME, **plus-size model**

New Shawls

Shawls in and of themselves, of course, aren't new. Your great-granny probably draped one over her shoulders to ward off the cold as she knitted your mom's booties on the front porch. What's new about today's shawls is their fabrics, their styling, and the actual way they're being worn. Modern shawls are often fringeless, multiseasonal, multioccasion, and come in many different wonderful fabrics—from featherweight chiffons and organzas

The important thing to remember is that covering up in fashion is much the same as covering up in politics: **You don't want anybody to notice that you're doing it!** So cover-ups shouldn't look like cover-ups. They should be subtle and stylish (probably a good policy for the political kind, too). A

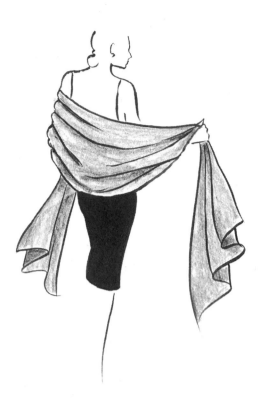

fancier shawls are perfect for evening. Aside from covering up, they finish off a bare evening dress beautifully and add a real touch of class. In cold weather, toss a cashmere or pashmina shawl over a jacket or coat for an extra layer of warmth.

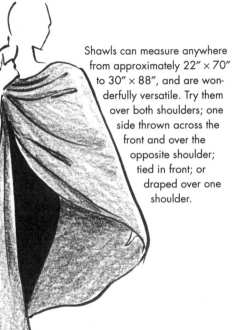

Shawls can measure anywhere from approximately 22" × 70" to 30" × 88", and are wonderfully versatile. Try them over both shoulders; one side thrown across the front and over the opposite shoulder; tied in front; or draped over one shoulder.

to silk, velvet, and cashmere. They're gorgeous! They add instant chic and softness and are just what the doctor ordered to put some pop in your monotones. Best of all, they make for artful camouflage.

Shawls, like scarves, are terrific for redirecting attention up and away from heavy hips and legs. They help balance bottom-heavy bodies by adding a little extra dimension on top, and they do a brilliant job of covering up dreaded bat wings, heavy upper arms, or simply undertoned arms. After all, not everybody has a personal trainer and sculpted arms like Angela Bassett or Madonna.

Even the sheerest, most diaphanous chiffon shawls can veil arms just enough to disguise imperfections, which makes them especially handy in summer when one part of you is dying to wear spaghetti-strap dresses and tube tops and the other part of you wouldn't dare. Woven linen and silk scarves are also terrific summer toppers. And

Think about shawls before you get rid of any questionable stuff in your closet, since they can cover a multitude of design sins and totally rejuvenate a terminally mediocre ensemble. Shawls also pack like a dream, making them ideal for travel, and here's the real topper—**they will always fit!** You can put on seven extra pounds tomorrow and your shawl will not be tight! They are unconditional in their support.

Plus, they are timeless. Shawls will not go out of style—in our lifetime anyway. They are classic fash-

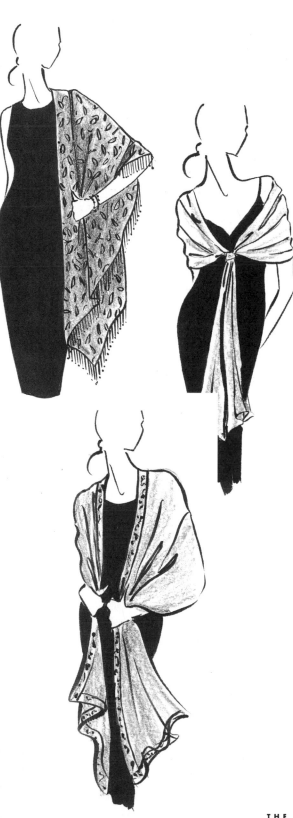

ion perennials. Sure, they may be more *la mode* one season than another, but they are simply too chic, practical, comfortable, and versatile to ever disappear entirely from the fashion scene. If you like wearing them, **get the best quality you can afford.** Luxury fabrics look luxurious. Should you ever tire of them, simply store them away for a year or so, and they will seem totally new and wonderful when you reintroduce them to your wardrobe. It will be like falling in love all over again . . . well, almost.

Scarves

Like shawls, superlarge, light-weight **square scarves** can also be used to cover upper arms. Fold into a triangle, wrap around the arms, and tie in front. Or try the "butterfly tie" with summer dresses. Fold the scarf in half, tie the ends together on each side, and slip your arms through the holes. Traditional smaller-sized square scarves are generally most effective at adding a dash of pizzazz and color and are good at keeping attention up around the face. **Oblong scarves, on the other hand, can actually cover up trouble spots as well.**

When you drape a long oblong around your neck and allow it to hang under an open jacket, for instance, it will drape right over your midriff and stomach, totally obscuring any problems in that area. Plus, it adds a very subtle sophisticated edge to the outfit. This works especially well if the scarf has some weight to it (but not bulk) and is in a contrasting texture, but the same color or tone, as the jacket. Example: a lush black, deep chocolate, or navy silk charmeuse scarf draped inside a black gabardine jacket. (See Rule 10 for the best ways to tie oblongs.)

One little warning: Don't try to use scarves to cover a short or thick neck—they will only make it look shorter or thicker.

Sarongs, Lungis, Pareos

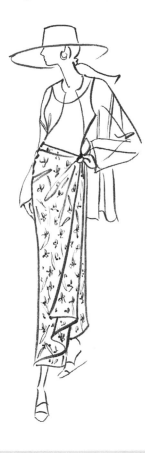

Scarves can look old-fashioned if they're tied around the head. But they don't if they're done in ample shapes to wear like a bandolier or pareo to tie over a pair of pants like a long skirt.

—GIORGIO ARMANI, designer

Sarongs (a.k.a. lungis and pareos) are almost as handy as shawls—at least in the summertime and in the tropics. **They're very effective cover-ups for heavyish hips and thighs, derrieres, and legs.** Plus, they're a natural at the beach or for hanging out, running errands, and other casual activities. You can even tie them over leggings or tights for a totally new look. They can also be worn shawl-like while sitting on the beach, to protect your skin from the sun.

I got hooked on them in Southeast Asia, where both men and women wear them for all occasions—and with nothing underneath! Here in the Western Hemisphere you might possibly want to wear underwear with them and are probably better off limiting their use to leisure wear—although who's to say you couldn't fashion a lovely silk lungi for evening? My friend Dina, a wardrobe supervisor, wears sarongs on the job all the time. She usually pairs hers with a T-shirt and a jean jacket and looks great. She, of course, is in L.A. *and* in showbiz. Obviously this is a very risky career look for a Chicago banker.

Back to the beach: The basic sarong is approximately 3½ feet wide and 5½ to 7 feet long. My favorites come from Indonesia, Thailand, and neighboring countries. They're made of a midweight cotton batik that has a decorative panel on one end, and they get softer and softer with each washing. (More expensive handmade batik is printed the same on both sides. Machine-printed batik has a right and wrong side.) Lighter-weight, thin cotton sarongs, which feel more like scarves, are more prevalent in the United States and touristy beach areas like the Caribbean. Some people find the lighter-weight material easier to wrap, but the batiks are just as easy after a little practice.

The right wrap is the real trick to wearing sarongs successfully. There are a slew of wrap variations to choose from. You might find that one variation stays put better on you than another, or that one wrap is more flattering or comfortable than another. So experiment with the following styles and see which you like best:

- *Caribbean beach wrap.* This is the easiest of all. It works best with soft scarf-like fabrics and needs a bathing suit underneath for modesty's sake. It can be tied high (above the bust) or low (on the hips). Simply grab the ends of the fabric, skinny them up a bit, and tie. Leave the ends hanging down to help cover the space where the two ends meet.

- *Caribbean dinner wrap.* This one provides full coverage and requires little to nothing underneath—and is formal enough to wear to a tropical moonlit dinner. Take the fabric behind you at the waist, leaving the right side longer than the left. Tie the end of the shorter left side to a little ear of fabric on the right, then wrap the rest of the right side around and across your front. Pull it snug and turn the top of the lungi over it.

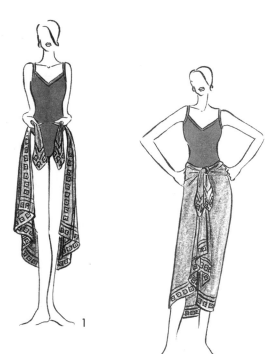

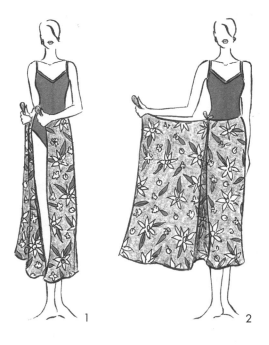
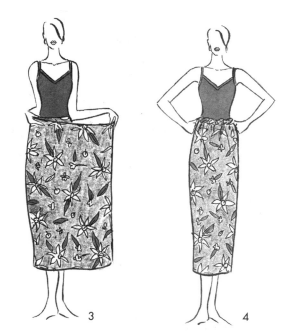

A variation: If the fabric is long enough, instead of tying the short piece to a little ear of fabric of the long piece, you can just wrap the long piece all the way around your body and tie it to the end of the short piece when they meet up.

• *Thai side wrap.* This is how women wrap their lungis in Thailand. Hold the fabric behind you at waist level, leaving the right side longer than the left (this is the border side if your fabric has one). Fold the short side across your front. Wind the top of the long side a bit, pull the short side snug against your body, then pull

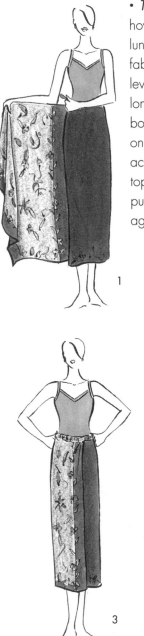

1

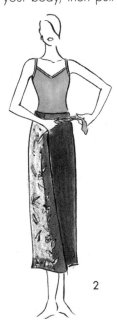

2

3

the longer, twisted side around your waist and tuck the top of the short side *over* the twisted part all around. (Can be tied above the bust as well.)

• *Burma (Myanmar) middle wrap.* The Burmese sew the ends of their lungis together with one seam to form a tube—no way to flip open, and great for modesty. The women wear it wrapped on the side similar to the Thai style. Men wrap it with a *middle fold,* which I find allows a much greater freedom of movement. Stand inside the tube with the border in the center (if there is one), hold up the middle close to your body, grab the edges of the tube, and crisscross

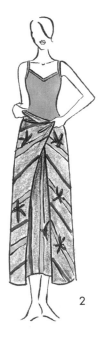

1

2

3

them over the center, twisting them together. Then fold the top of the fabric over all around. You should have a nice inverted pleat in the front.

There is really no end to the ways you can tie lungis, so get creative. The other night I saw a woman at a party who had wrapped one as a dress. She looked great, but I couldn't for the life of me figure out how she had wrapped the thing. When I asked her, she said she really didn't know, she and her roommate had just played around until it looked right.

> *They look great on people of all shapes. . . . Sometimes you just don't feel like walking around in a bikini letting it all hang out.*
>
> —KATHY IRELAND, model, on sarongs

Artful Layering

Layering is one of the best cover-up techniques going. Sometimes all it takes is one extra little layer to make a tummy disappear, to skinny up the hips, or rebalance your proportions. Once you get into it and let your imagination loose, you'd be surprised at the combinations you can come up with. Some ideas to get you started:

DOUBLING UP ON SIMILAR SHAPES

This essentially means wearing two tops of relatively lightweight material that are very close in shape and design. You could, for instance, wear two silk blouses, tuck the bottom one in, leave the top one partially unbuttoned, and wear it as a sort of shirt jacket that would cover waistline, midriff, and tummy. Pop the collar of the underblouse over

the outerblouse collar and give the sleeves a roll. If the outerblouse were a nice darkish neutral and the underblouse were a bright or light neutral, you'd be getting a twofer: The color would direct attention to the face, and the shirt jacket would mask any imperfections in the torso and help form a slimming vertical line as it blended in with the dark neutral bottom.

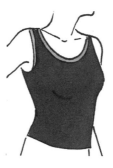

You could get a similar effect with a longer, larger (dark) tank top over a smaller (lighter) one. The light one underneath would peek out in the front around the neckline and straps, bringing interest up to the face, while the darker one would keep the silhouette slim as it falls gracefully over the stomach and waist. In this scenario you also have the added bonus of an extra layer to keep your bra from showing through the tight lighter-colored top.

TIERING

Tiering is a variation of the doubling-up theme. Here, though, the under layer is longer than the top layer (see picture). This sort of **tiered effect** can be extremely slimming when done well. Suggestions: First, stick with the same colors or tones. If the under layer is too much of a contrast, you can end up with an attention-grabbing horizontal stripe where you don't want it. Second, shapes must be slim and cut in a way that they skim the body—sort of float just around it. And third, fabrics must be lightweight, soft, and drapey. Slightly transparent tops worn over opaque ones are another terrific look—although a wee bit trendy.

JACKETS

We've gotten so used to wearing jackets that, like the old friends they are, we take them for granted. But they are in fact an excellent camouflager and indispensable when it comes to layering, since they're cross-seasonal and look great with almost anything from leggings and jeans to dresses and skirts.

Jackets *can* **camouflage pretty much every-thing**—bust, arms, hips, waist, derriere, and upper thighs. Whether they actually *do* or not depends on the styles and cuts you pick. **Jacket cuts** pretty much boil down to fitted, semifitted, and unconstructed. Style detailing includes length, lapel shape, pocket placement, etc.

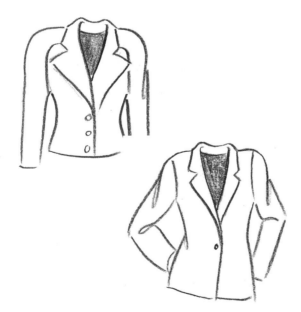

If you remember to stick to vertical lines, keep it simple, and watch your balance (Rules 3, 12, and 4, respectively), you'll automatically choose the right styles. A short fitted jacket, which makes the top look smaller, for instance, would obviously not be a good choice for a full-hipped/slender-shouldered woman, since her balance discrepancy would then be emphasized. She would be better balanced in a fitted to semi-fitted cut with good shoulders that is midhip length to long. A top-heavy/slim-hipped woman has more options. As long as she keeps her hips looking slim and good vertical lines in her jacket, she'll be fine. As for women with large derrieres, one of the best looks is a dress or a skirt that falls perfectly straight over the rear covered by a shortish jacket that ends just where the rear starts (good tailoring is crucial for this one).

But even if a jacket is an ideal style for your body shape, what you wear with your jacket makes a huge—*repeat, huge*—difference in how slimming it is on you. In general, shorter jackets are best with fuller slacks or skirts and longer jackets with narrower pants and skirts. But even so, very slight variations can make a difference. Case in point: My favorite jacket of all time is a black mandarin collar Emanuel. It looks terrific with slim pants—which is what I usually wear—so I've worn that jacket to death. But it *adds* pounds to my figure when I try it on with narrow skirts—of any length—or with my new favorite calf-length tube dress. It's simply too long and not narrow enough. Yet it looks perfectly narrow with the slim pants. This is not proportion nit-picking—which I admit I'm wont to do. Even my husband notices the difference. Luckily, I recently found an ultranarrow DKNY one-button black jacket that looks incredible with both the tube dress and the skirts. The moral is this: **You have to try jackets on with what you intend to wear them with. They** *won't* **look the same with everything.**

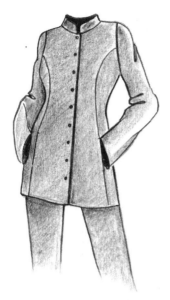

In general, the simpler the jacket—that is, the cleaner the lines, the fewer the buttons and design details—the better. A jacket that is cut well doesn't need embellishment to make it work. **Moral: Trust the cut.**

CAMISOLES

Camisoles are wonderful first layers under almost everything—blouses, jackets, dresses, you name it.

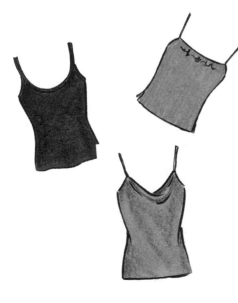

VESTS

Vests are a natural for layering and are great for concealing major torso problems. Here, length, texture, and cut are what count.

Long, unfitted duster vests: You've seen this one if you were a fan of TV's *Maude*—it was Bea Arthur's signature look. Worn full length or below the hips, these soft, unstructured layers can help camouflage hips, stomachs, and waists. You can pop them over almost any kind of top: T-shirts, blouses, camisoles, etc. Dusters hang straight from the shoulders and are usually worn open, providing nice long vertical lines on each side of the body. The ones that are cut a little narrower on top will generally be more flattering. One thing about these kinds of vests: they truly work only in knits, jerseys, heavy silks, and other *soft* fabrics that move with the body yet are weighty enough not to cling to it. Stiff fabrics look big and boxy. If you're short, you'll probably be better off with the shorter vests.

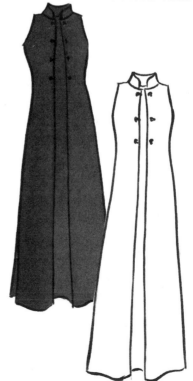

Short vests are brilliant at neutralizing bust size, concealing thick waists and belly rolls, and lengthening short waists. They can be worn closed or open, fitted or narrow, and fall just below the waist or to the hipbone. Since they don't require as much movement as long, unfitted vests, they look fine in linen and other less fluid (but not stiff!) fabrics. Watch the shape of the vest bottoms—styles that have slightly V-shaped bottoms are often more flattering than ones that go straight across (love those verticals). Also, try layering them *over* longer tops for a slightly newer look.

CARDIGAN SWEATERS

Cardigans are perfect for layering and wonderfully versatile. Long slim ones create a nice long vertical line when paired with slim pants or a straight skirt, as well as covering hips, backsides, and waist dimension. Cardigans that hit at the hipbone, or a little below, disguise thick waists and tummy bulges, and help lengthen a short waist. The best shapes in both cases are slim, with no binding on the bottom—all binding does is create a lethal horizontal line at precisely the wrong place. Whether cardigans are cashmere, cotton, linen, crochet, or something in between, make sure the fabric has enough weight and body to hang well, so that it doesn't cling to your body.

Some ways to wear your cardigans:

• **Open as a jacket** over another top—long ones cover the hips and rear and disguise waists.

• **Buttoned halfway up over a T-shirt, tank, or camisole**—creates an elongating V neck. Covers tummy, waist, upper hips. Works in either long or hipbone length.

• **Buttoned up the back under a shirt or jacket.** Hipbone length is best for this one.

• **Over a little summer frock**—covers arms.

• **Tied around your shoulders**—brings interest to the face.

• **Tied around your waist**—covers up your derriere and tummy. Any length will work.

• **Tied across your body.** I've humbly named this one after myself since I wear my sweaters like this all the time—and hey, I'm writing the book. So here's how you do the *Leah Feldon wrap:* Swing your sweater over your shoulders as if you were going to tie it in front, then drop one sleeve under your arm and tie it to the sleeve coming over the other shoulder. It adds a certain *je ne sais quoi* to your entire outfit. Plus it holds buttonless jackets closed.

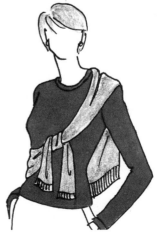

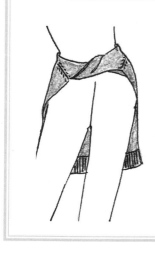

Diana Vreeland had the waist tie totally down—although she actually *wrapped* more than tied. After she had her cashmere (always cashmere) cardigan perfectly adjusted across her backside, she'd take the sleeves around front and intertwine them just so, tucking the sleeve ends up and under. There were never any sleeves dangling. The look is still a winner!

CARDIGAN/JACKET HYBRIDS

As the name suggests, these are sort of like jackets and sort of like cardigans. They're shaped like cardigans and are made of woven fabrics as well as knits. But they have nontraditional cardigan necklines, such as notched collars, V necks, or even mandarin collars, and occasionally have detailing like little pockets. They're a terrific cardigan alternative.

SHIRTS AND TUNICS

Relaxed-fit big shirts and tunics that button down the front are good versatile pieces for layering, since you can wear them as shirt jackets as well. Side slits add movement. Make sure the twenty-nine-inch standard length isn't too long for you.

DUSTERS AND COATS

Full-length dusters and coats are also contenders, as long as they drape well and don't overwhelm your figure.

FOUR GOOD GENERAL LAYERING RULES TO KEEP IN MIND

- Layer with lightweight fabrics that drape.
- Keep the first layer snug.
- Add color underneath, rather than on top.
- Except for the snug underlayer, layers should skim, not cling.

BEWARE OF STIFF, SHINY, OR BULKY FABRICS

> Now, what is this padded thing? Are you crazy to think women are going to wear a padded skirt? They're hideous. I look obese. And if I put this on and look obese, what about women with curves?
>
> —GWYNETH PALTROW
> . . . on a very short-lived trend

The other day, I was flipping through an old issue of *InStyle*, and I was mystified by a little snippet I found. It was in a section called "The Look." Now, for those of you who do not regularly indulge in the joyous voyeuristic pleasures of *InStyle*, this is where the editors compile pictures of similarly clad celebrities and chat up the resulting montage as a fabulous new minitrend. In this particular instance, the trend was siren wraps, and they were exalting the glories of "short sleek coats in some stiff, shiny fabric"!

Well, my jaw just about hit the floor. Stiff, shiny fabrics sleek? I don't think so! Not only do stiff fabrics make you look fat, but shiny ones can too. And together they're about as gruesome as it gets. I couldn't help but wonder what those savvy trendsetters at *InStyle* were thinking. Didn't they notice that all five celebrities pictured looked considerably less than sleek in their new siren wraps?

The Following Textures Can Be Hazardous to Your Figure

STIFF

Garments made from **stiff** fabrics tend to disregard your shape and take on one of their own—which is likely to be square and boxy, like the *InStyle* siren wraps mentioned above. Cube, I feel confident in saying, is not a shape most of us are craving. The other major shape created by stiff fabrics is big and contrived, like Scarlett O'Hara's curtain dress or a fifties poodle skirt. The only time I've seen stiff work, at least in this decade, is in big-skirted formal attire and wedding dresses—and even then there was always a certain softness to the material. So it's pretty safe to say that stiff fabrics will make you look larger than you want to. Stiff is a good texture for tents, not clothes.

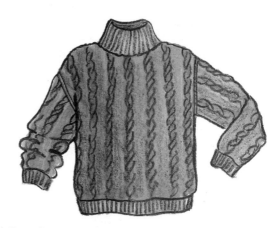

Stiff is also a texture that can pop up in almost every kind of material made, since its presence is more dependent on how the yarn is made, woven, and finished than on the fiber itself. Thus, any fiber—wool, cotton, linen, synthetics, even silk—can produce some stiff textures. Since content labels won't give you a clue about the stiffness of a garment, you have to rely on your senses to literally feel it out. You have to handle it, try it on, and move around in it. **The bottom line: If it feels stiff it *is* stiff—even if it is 100 percent silk or cashmere.** It's one of those walk like a duck, talk like a duck things.

Obviously, some garments will be less fluid than others. A pair of jeans or cotton flat-front pants, for example, will be stiffer than a pair of double-ply silk pajama pants. A summer linen jacket will be crisper than one in silk crêpe. But even in those cases, *softer is better.*

BULKY

Bulky fabrics simply add mass. They can, depending on the exact fabric and cut of the garment, add more than an inch to your frame all around. Picture the thickness of a fisherman's sweater, heavy corduroy slacks, or a hand-knit ski sweater, for example. That thickness transfers to *you* as soon as you put on the garment. Instant weight gain! In addition to nubby tweeds, heavy knits, and corduroys, watch the thickness of velvets, chenilles, and flannels. Always go for the finer, lighter-weight variety. Newer, sportier fabrics like polar fleece are extremely lightweight and practical. I love them for

fall and winter coats and jackets. But they really bulk you up when they're made into pants and *some* tops. So watch it!

Don't let this bulky fabric alert prod you into overcompensating with paper-thin fabrics. With the exception perhaps of sheer diaphanous fabrics like chiffon and summer linens, fabrics must have enough weight to fall naturally without clinging. *This is essential!* Nothing is tackier than cheap thin fabric that shows every ripple of flesh and underwear, or that sticks to your thighs when you move. Nice weighty tights with a good percentage of Lycra will make you look two sizes smaller than a cheap flimsy pair. Same for stretchy tops (should you venture into that territory). Even a simple T-shirt looks better in a nice heavyweight cotton.

SHINY

With **shiny** textures, it's the reflective surface that makes you look bigger. Instead of absorbing light like matte textures do, the light bounces off the fabric, optically enlarging both you and the garment. The reflected light also highlights every little crease in the fabric and, when the garment is snug, outlines even the most minuscule bump on your body—a tiny postdinner belly bulge, a mosquito bite on your bum. So think twice about how you wear satin, sequins, taffeta, charmeuse, velvet, leather, and metallics. A little bit of shiny—say a silk charmeuse shell or scarf under a jacket, a sequined top, a beaded lapel on a matte jacket, or a satin shawl—all this is fine and can, in fact, make for a wonderfully interesting texture mix. But all-over shine—a long Jean Harlow satin gown, a form-fitting Lurex dress, a gold lamé pants suit, or even silk charmeuse pajamas—will make for a bigger, albeit *chatoyante*, you.

Rule of thumb: The shinier the fabric, the bigger the risk. The more matte, the safer you are. Deep-pile fabrics like velvet and chenille reflect light but considerably less light than satin. Some terrific silks and synthetics have **more *sheen* than *shine*** to them. Choose garments made from these "semi-gloss" fabrics with a very discriminating eye. When in doubt, do without. Leather jackets are borderline—they may be acceptable if the cut is exquisite, but puleeeeeeze never wear them with tight leather pants!

FLUFFY, FEATHERY, FUZZY, AND FURRY

These speak for themselves. What's the point? They just add more unnecessary bulk. Give away your cuddly fuzzy angora sweaters, boas, and fake furs. *Somebody will just love them!*

> *The worst time for fashion was the late eight-ies: the bulky shoulder pads, the Dynasty-inspired evening gowns with tacky beading.*
>
> —RICHARD TYLER, designer

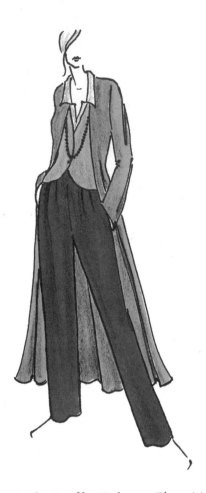

The Right Stuff—Fabrics That Move!

Movement and *drape* are the key words here. They're the qualities that make clothes look graceful and elegant—and make you look slimmer. The most flattering and most chic clothes skim your body and move *with* you, rather than standing out aloofly on their own. Picture yourself walking in a soft, fluid skirt that falls in slimming vertical lines around your body. Then picture the same stride in a rigid A-line style. There's no contest. Even tailored jackets, which you may not particularly think of as having movement, actually do when made out of a soft, fluid fabric that allows drape.

Fabrics that drape and move well are usually a better quality and as such can cost more. All I can say is, it's worth the difference. Shop the sales and outlet malls if need be, but don't compromise on fabric. Even a great design can look totally bargain basement if it's made from a cheap, inflexible fabric.

> I like clothes that are feminine and have movement in them. They make me look long and lean.
>
> —PRISCILLA PRESLEY, actress

If there's the least doubt in your mind what I mean when I talk about movement, you owe it to yourself to drop by the most exclusive shop in your area where you can try on couture-quality clothing. It doesn't matter whether you can afford it or not, trying on is free! Pick out the two-thousand-dollar Armani jacket or the five-thousand-dollar Givenchy gown and consciously pay attention to the feel or *hand* of the fabric—and watch the way it moves and drapes. For this particular experiment, stick to the more classic designers like Armani, Michael Kors, Calvin Klein, Ralph Lauren, and Donna Karan, all of whom have an affinity for fine fabrics. Some of the trendier, more avant-garde designers seem to find the seventies retro polyester thing amusing at the moment—there's not a lot to learn there.

> Evening wear is at its most modern when it combines simple shapes with evocative materials.
>
> —MARK BADGLEY AND JAMES MISCHKA, designers

Fabric: Facts and Favorites

Since I've noted some general fabric confusion in my workshops, you might be feeling it, too. So let me give you my ten-cent fabric miniprimer. Everyone should know this—a well-informed consumer, after all, is a good consumer.

There are *four basic natural fibers* that go way back to ancient times—wool, silk, linen, and cotton—which can all be blended with one another. Then there's rayon (first made in 1884) and more recently lyocell (trade name Tencel), which could be considered "new naturals" since they're derived from wood cellulose, as opposed to chemicals. And then there are the *synthetics* (polyesters et al.), which are whipped up in labs. And finally there are *synthetic blends*—marriages of a natural with a synthetic. *Fiber,* then, is your base material.

What you *do* with the fiber—the type of yarn you make from it and how you weave that yarn—is what gives a fabric its generic name. Which is why you hear cotton also being referred to as percale, ticking, terry cloth, jersey, velour, broadcloth, muslin, canvas, seersucker, chambray, cheesecloth, denim, gabardine, serge, corduroy, and chenille, just to name a few of its incarnations. It's also why fabrics such as crêpe, gabardine, velvet, poplin, batiste, etc., are not all alike. Two gabardines, for instance, may have been *woven* in the same manner, but they have different qualities when made from different *fibers.*

That said—a few Camouflage Chic favorites:

• *Gabardine:* A lightweight, finely woven twill fabric with very fine diagonal ridges, which looks totally smooth and drapes *extremely* well. Lightweight wool gabardine is a wonderful multiseasonal fabric, perfect for suits, jackets, skirts, and pants. *A great choice for wardrobe basics.* Gab also works well in silk, cotton, rayon, and quality man-mades.

- **Crêpe:** A plain-weave matte fabric with a slightly crinkly surface. It resists wrinkling and drapes wonderfully in wool. Also a winner in silk and rayon. Works beautifully in most styles.

- **Knits:** The best knits for sweaters and cardigans are cashmere and merino wool. For dresses and skirts, you need a heavier wool knit. If a knit is cut close to the body, it will cling and you will have to be in a skinny phase to wear it. Generally best as a first layer.

- **Jersey:** A lightweight fine knit. Wonderful in soft cotton, silk, wool, rayon, and linen. *Terrific for layering.* Nothing beats a fine cotton jersey T-shirt or dress in summer.

- **Silk charmeuse:** A smooth, heavy, dressy, shiny silk. Okay, it's shiny, but it's great for blouses and camisoles under jackets and for scarves. Adds richness and texture.

- **Silk—smooth or washed:** Look for two- to four-ply silk, which will give you the best drape. For trousers, stick to four-ply whenever possible.

- **Rayon** (a.k.a. *viscose*) **and Tencel** (a.k.a. *lyocell*)**:** Allow for great drape. Look for fabrics with a nice medium weight, good hand, and substantial body. Good for skirts, loose pants, tops, and unstructured jackets.

- **Synthetics:** There are still natural-fiber snobs out there who won't go near a man-made fiber. But as far as I'm concerned, if something feels great and looks great and just happens to be man-made, it doesn't matter. In fact, the label inside one of my very favorite jackets reads 100 percent polyester. Synthetics keep getting better and better, and these days so many good designers are using them that sooner or later they're probably going to end up on your body. In the long run, you have to judge synthetics as you do all fabrics—by the feel and touch. Some *microfibers*, which are basically very finely woven synthetic fibers, have a wonderful feel and actually breathe, too. It's a brave new material world.

- **Lycra.** Since I've probably mentioned Lycra at least ten times already, I thought I'd better give the official word on what it is exactly. Lycra is DuPont's trademarked name for spandex. Spandex is simply a stretchy elastic synthetic fiber, which has, for the most part, replaced rubber in the clothing industry.

> [To resist synthetics] is like saying, "I don't want to work on a computer."
>
> —DONNA KARAN, **designer**

RULE 8

BUILD ON THE RIGHT FOUNDATIONS

Shapewear is essentially soft, pliable, pretty underwear—heavily dosed with Lycra—that is designed to trim, slim, and mold. It can take inches off in various strategic places without killing you or rearranging your ribs—always a plus. There are designs that can trim your thighs, flatten your belly, whittle your middle, lift your derriere, contour your bust, and generally slim you down and eliminate jiggle. And that, needless to say, can make a huge difference in how you look in your clothes—and how you feel in them, for that matter. You'll obviously move with more confidence knowing that everything is firmly in place and your behind doesn't look like "two ferrets fighting in a bag" (this is the ever-colorful duchess of York's description, not mine).

> *The truth is that every woman thinks she sees a bulge, even when there isn't necessarily one there.*
>
> —NANCY GANZ, shapewear designer

First there was underwear. Now there is "shapewear." Well, I suppose there always was shapewear if you count stomachers, farthingales, whalebone corsets, rubber girdles, etc. But really, those ancient contraptions were more "torturewear" than anything else. It took centuries of going through the hoops—or tripping over them, anyway—to get us into today's new painless shapewear.

How Comfortable Is Shapewear?

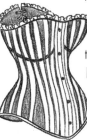

The comfort factor is purely subjective. It depends on how you feel about *tight.* If you're a little claustrophobic and usually wear very loose, unconstructed clothing, it'll be a stretch for you—both literally and figuratively. If you're perfectly content in panty hose, sports bras, and workout gear, it shouldn't be a big deal—shapewear's just the next step. In my informal, absolutely scientifically imprecise survey, one woman described wearing a full-length body slip as "comforting, like being gently held"; another claimed a waist cincher improved her posture and alleviated back pain; and another reported feeling "confined and restricted" in both gizmos. The bottom line: **You have to try it for yourself.**

Almost all intimate apparel companies have some shapewear in their lines— some more than others. Donna Karan Intimates, for instance, has about seven stylish pieces in its Bodywear line, including its top-selling "contour bicycle pants." Strouse, Adler's Smoothie line offers a good comprehensive collection of Body Re-formers, one-piece ultracontrol bodysuits and slips, as well as Tummy Terminators and Waist Eliminators. Playtex has, among other things, a good selection of pretty tummy-toning panties in its Secrets and Eighteen Hour lines—the latter geared toward bigger women. Wacoal offers several styles of moderate to firm control panties, briefs, and long-leg styles. Wonderbra has enticing body suits and control slips. Maidenform covers the gamut with its Flex-ees line. Olga, Josie Natori . . . even Oscar de la Renta is in on the act. And the list goes on.

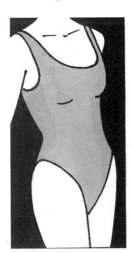

One of the most fashion-forward lines is arguably Bodyslimmers by Nancy Ganz. Nancy, a former sportswear designer, keeps a keen eye on fashion trends and is always there to support them with young, hip, sexy new designs. When asymmetrical gowns were hot, for instance, Bodyslimmers was on the spot with one-shoulder camisoles and body slips. And it now offers, among other things, a couple of ultraslenderizing body slips that could make wearing some of those seriously formfitting, models-only dresses an actual possibility—should you dare.

What Does What to What

Now for specifics. Here's a sampling of what's available and what it can do for your various and sundry parts:

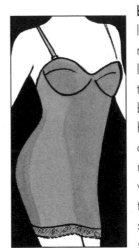

• **For torsos:** The aforementioned **body slips** and **bodysuits.** These make for long slim lines, eliminating midriff bulge, little potbellies, and underwear lines at the waist and under the bust. Most snap or have hooks and eyes at the crotch. Available in a range of styles, from those with underwire demi-bra tops with removable straps—great for tube tops, strapless gowns, and other adventuresome attire—to tank tops. Perfect under knits and matte jersey. Also excellent as a first layer under sheers.

• **For hips: Bodysuits, body slips, half-slips.** The stretchy, body-molding Hipslip was Nancy Ganz's first foray into shapewear territory— and she built an empire on it. It works! It tames tummy bulges, shirt rumples, hip ripples and jiggles. Nancy's comes with a built-in thong to

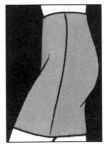

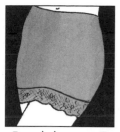

eliminate dreaded VPL (visible panty lines). Flexees and Smoothie also have excellent versions on the market. Body slips and bodysuits will also slim hips.

- **For abdomens: Tummy-toner panties.** While they won't give you a washboard cut, they can give you back your flat stomach (if it's not too far gone). I personally road-tested Nancy's Bellybuster brief and her Waist Cincher panty, both of which I found comfortable and effective—and I liked the high-cut leg that kept them from looking like panty girdles. Mainstream companies generally cut a little more conservatively—a good choice if you need more coverage. Lots of choices in this area.

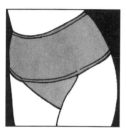 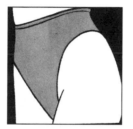

- **For midriffs: Waist cinchers, bodysuits, body slips.** Nancy's Hi-Waisted Bellybuster is especially effective. Also check out Flexees Waist Nipper brief and control slip, Donna Karan's Bodywear midriff pant, and Smoothie's Waist Eliminator.

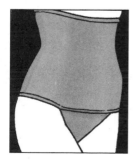

- **For rear ends: Derriere lifters** boost your behind while smoothing over tummy bulge and hip blips. Nancy says her Butt Booster "truly defies gravity." Derriere lifters are also available from both Flexees and Playtex.

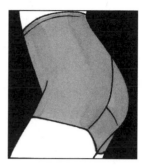

- **For legs: Long-leg panties** for thighs. Every manufacturer has some form of this traditional girdle shape. Bodyslimmers takes it to an art with its Hi-Waisted Thighslimmer, which cinches the midriff *and* trims the thigh all the way to the knee. Also from Bodyslimmers is the Legliner—essentially a Lycra heavy-control legging (it took my leg down a size). "Renovator" is Strouse, Adler's version of the control legging. Also try workout compression shorts—a good non-panty-hose alternative for women whose thighs tend to rub together in summer.

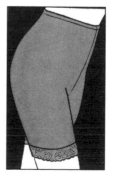 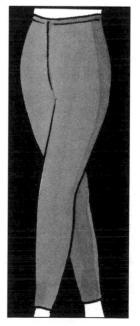

And that, my friends, is the shapewear story. For the moment, anyway. It is ever changing, so stay tuned. It's up to you whether or not you hop on the bandwagon. With loose-fitting clothes, shapewear will probably be totally unnecessary, and some days you might just want to let it all hang out. But on the days when you need a little help, at least you know it's there. Most top department stores carry a good selection of shapewear these days. (If you have trouble finding Bodyslimmers, call 1-800-426-SLIP for the store nearest you.)

Basic Underwear

Shapewear aside, even your choices of regular-type underwear can make a big difference in how you look in clothes. Undergarments are truly the foundation of your wardrobe. If the foundation is shaky (literally, yet again), your whole look can fall apart. So your regular stuff has to be the right stuff. **Good underwear should fit, flatter, and be garment appropriate.**

> *All those lines and ridges distort a girl.*
>
> —MARILYN MONROE, actress,
> on why she wore no underwear

PANTIES

If your panty lines are generally visible, it's time to rethink your panty styles. **Visible panty lines** are not a good look. Aside from being plain unsightly, they often create bulges that make you look fat. **Bikinis** are especially deadly because they create lines and bumps across the buttocks *and* on the hips, which draws attention to what many women would consider an undesirable focus spot. The VPLs have to go.

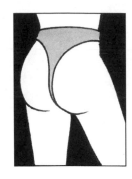

So what to do? Some shapewear, such as the Thighslimmer and Hipslip mentioned above, are terrific solutions. Panty hose are another good alternative. And then there's **the thong.** A thong, for those of you who have had your head buried in books or babies for the last decade, is a pair of panties without a back. Well, actually there is a back, but not much of one—just a ribbon-wide piece of material that tucks between your buttocks and sort of disappears—a very fashionable look on Rio beaches.

If you've never worn thong panties, here's the deal: To look good in them without clothes on, you really need one of those firm, sculpted bottoms most of us could only get with an airbrush. But with your clothes on, you can be way less than perfect—it really doesn't matter. **Thongs give you an incredibly smooth look under pants, body-hugging skirts, leggings, bike shorts, workout togs, etc.** There's not a panty line in sight! Seamless! Since most styles come up to the waist in the front, they're totally smooth across the stomach too. Plus, if the Lycra content is high they can even help hold in your tummy.

As for comfort, well, that's sort of an acquired taste—like caviar. You have to get used to them. Some women do and some don't. I personally avoided thongs for years because they just looked so annoying. I always thought they would be a constant irritant, like a pebble in a shoe. Recently, though, when I couldn't take seeing the panty lines in my leggings anymore, I bought a couple pair of thongs and gave them a try. It turns out they're not as bad as I thought—more a presence really than a discomfort. I'm still not totally sold on them for every day, but they make my bum look so much better in pants and tights that I'm hoping one day I'll reach the point where I'll come to fully accept them and we will become one. The Zen of Thong.

A few tips:

- Try tummy-toners for everyday. The lightweight variety has less Lycra overall, so they're less restricting while still effective.

- Bikini wearers—if you're in for a little more coverage and fewer lines, try your favorite style one size *bigger*.

- Forget about boy legs—you know, the ones that go straight across the top of the thigh. They really look best on boys—and prepubescent girls. If you have any meat on your thighs, they'll just bind and make ridges. Very unattractive.

PANTY HOSE

Panty hose have come a long way. They're doing things with microfiber these days that make them al-

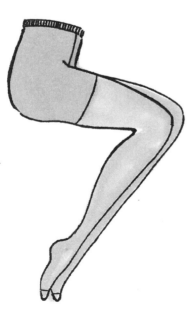

most cozy and much more comfortable than they used to be. They're still a pain to get into, but I don't hate them as much as I used to. The way I feel about panty hose is this: **If you have to wear them, they might as well make you look skinnier.**

Most good hosiery companies have lines specifically designed for extra control. Some take it to an art. Shock Up by Oroblu (made in Italy) is the crème de la crème. It's not only designed to slim the waist, hips, and tummy *and* boost the derriere (it promises "to do for a woman's bottom what the push-up bra did for her breasts"!) but is also "enhanced with a 'massaging' leg with graded compression to slim, reduce fatigue, and energize." I personally road-tested a pair, and I have to admit they pretty much worked as advertised. My bottom was definitely boosted, my stomach was flatter and my legs trimmer. (I didn't wear them long enough to get energized.) Shock Ups could shake you up at thirty dollars a pop. But at least they're guaranteed for eight wearings, so they might, in the long run, be worth it—at least for those special times when you need a special boost. (Shock Ups are available at Saks, Nordstrom, Neiman-Marcus, Bloomingdale's, and specialty boutiques.) For every day, a good midrange (approximately nine dollars) body-contouring hose like Hanes Smooth Illusions might suit you just fine. The feel is slightly less luxurious and the control not quite as ultra, but it is still very impressive. Both these styles, and most other serious contouring hose, have a color definition line where the control panty stops and the sheer stockings begin, so they are not recommended for micro-minis.

In the light-control, sheer-to-the-waist category I love Oroblu Repos and Donna Karan Evolution. I found them both very cozy. They *do* look fabulous with minis. They're support compression hose that massage, support, and slim the leg, but look amazingly sheer.

BRAS

You must have the right bra. The wrong bra can make big women look bigger and all women look pretty shabby. The two major considerations with a bra are *style* and **fit.**

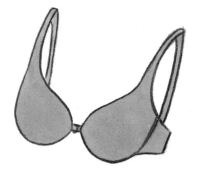

Style: Stylewise, your bra has to be compatible with your outfit. This may sound rather obvious, but it's easy to get so used to whatever style you're wearing that it doesn't even occur to you to switch for specific garments. Some women, for instance, are so addicted to their sexy push-up bras that they're blind to the fact that the bras look rather odd under snug knits. So for the record: push-up bras are designed to raise the breast up out of the bra on top to create cleavage—a sexy look in a low-cut top. Under knits, jerseys, and other close-fitting fabrics, however, what you get is decidedly *unsexy* lumps on top of the breasts. Textured, lacy bras are not well suited to knits either. **A bra with perfectly seamless molded cups is a best bet for body-conscious tops,** since nipples won't show through and it looks extremely natural under most garments. It's a good candidate for your everyday bra.

Other style tips:

• For some of your more esoteric clothing consider *specialty bras.* Smoothie has some very handy three-in-one convertible bra styles in its line. They can be worn with their straps set wide, criss-crossed across the back, or halter style—which is ideal for backless dresses. It also has a model with four-way convertible straps that does all the above plus comes together in the back like a racer-back style, which is perfect for tops that are cut out at the shoulders.

• Aside from strapless bras, there are a plethora of **bustier styles** around for strapless gowns and dresses. Donna Karan's bandeau bra is terrific for tube tops.

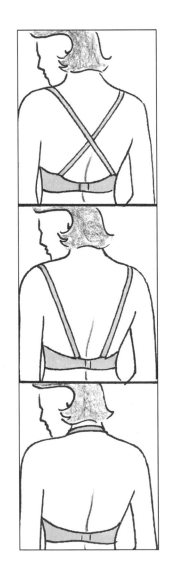

- For best support, try **underwire styles** (the curved wires underneath the breasts should be well padded for comfort). This style also lifts and shapes—highly recommended for you full-figured gals.

- **Front-closure styles,** which hook between the breasts, eliminate hook bumps on the back. The only drawback is that they are less size adjustable, because there's only one hook position. It's a trade-off.

- **Padded bras** are still a viable choice for small-busted women who need a little extra dimension to balance their figures.

- Bras with **side support panels** are an excellent choice for women who tend to bulge on the sides under the arms. The panels ease breasts forward for a sleeker, more natural look.

- Extra-large-busted women should consider **minimizer bras,** which do just the opposite of side-panel styles. They reduce the size of large breasts by shifting breast tissue from the front to the sides. Also look for padded straps for extra comfort.

- A lightly lined **contour bra** is a good idea when you want to camouflage nipples under sheer tops.

- **Cami-bras** are fun hybrids—bras with tops that look like camisoles when they peek out of your blouse.

Fit: Experts figure that 70 percent of us wear the wrong size bra, so there's a good chance that number includes you. Bodies change with weight gain or loss, childbirth, illness, exercise, age, and probably a zillion other things. So if you've been wearing the same size bra for the last two years (what? did you say more?), it would probably be a good idea to get refitted. Most good department stores have pros who not only know about fit but are also familiar with all the different brands and styles available. Call ahead to make sure there's a trained fitter on the premises; if there is, schedule an appointment. If the store doesn't have a fitter, try another store or ask if it has any upcoming fit events scheduled. I know that Playtex conducts workshops from time to time. And Wacoal has teams of specialists visiting stores across the country with its Silhouette Analyzer, a digital imaging computer that draws outlines of your silhouette in both your current bra and one chosen by its experts. There are bound to be other companies sponsoring similar programs. These kinds of workshops are always free, so if you have the time, you might as well take advantage of them.

FIT FORMULA

Simply measure all the way around just above your breasts for band size: i.e., 36 inches equals a size-36 bra. For cup size, measure across the fullest part of your breasts. Then subtract the band size from that number. Each additional inch represents a cup size. A one-inch difference is an A, two inches a B, three inches a C, etc.

Determining your size: Until you get to a fitter, try the following fit formula to determine your bra size. But also keep in mind that one manufacturer's 34B is often another's 34C. In fact, there are even size variations in different lines by the same company. So use the fit formula below as a guideline to get you in the right ballpark, so to speak—then try on every bra in the house.

Telltale signs that your bra doesn't fit properly:

• It hurts. It's supposed to be comfortable.

• You have bulges on the top or the sides of the cup.

• The cup puckers.

• The bra rides up in the back.

• The center of the bra doesn't lie flat against your breastbone.

• The straps dig into your shoulders or slip off your shoulders.

Bra Alternatives: If you're relatively small-busted you can get by with a bra alternative. Try body slips (great for under sheer dresses), bodysuits, tank tops, undershirts, tube tops, bandeau tops, or camisoles.

Intimate apparel manufacturers are coming up with new designs all the time. So if you haven't shopped for lingerie in a while—other than just zipping in to buy your standard undies—drop by your favorite store for a consultation. It might help you get in good shape.

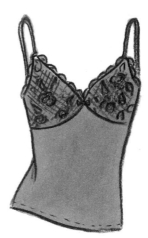

DON'T LET YOUR ACCESSORIES BRING YOU DOWN

> Boots and shoes are the greatest trouble of my life. Everything else one can turn and turn about, and make old look like new; but there's no coaxing boots and shoes to look better than they are.
>
> —GEORGE ELIOT, English novelist

> I'm always more comfortable underdressed than over. . . . I'm finding no jewelry very refreshing.
>
> —MICHELLE PFEIFFER, actress

SHOES

Women make more mistakes in their choice of shoes than any other accessory. Some of that might have to do with comfort—it's tricky to find shoes that look fabulous and are comfortable. But more often than not, it's simply a matter of choosing unsuitable styles—which not only can make you look shorter and heavier but can change the entire mood and attitude of your outfit as well.

Case in point: A few years ago Pamela Anderson Lee was on *Live! With Regis and Kathie Lee*. She was pregnant at the time and had on a cute little floral summer dress. Had she worn espadrilles, sandals, or little flats with the dress, she would have looked like a nice, pretty, wholesome girl next door, the Hollywood version of someone you wouldn't mind your brother dating. But Pamela opted for knee-high, high-heeled, white patent leather boots and ended up looking . . . well, I

You wouldn't think an innocent little thing like a simple accessory could thwart your attempts at slimness, but then nobody thought the *Titanic* would sink, either. The truth is that your choice of shoes, hosiery, belts, scarves, jewelry, etc. can make or break you. Let's cut right to the chase and start with shoes since they are major culprits in the "break you" department.

don't want to say *trashy* exactly, but I'm stuck for a more appropriate word. These boots, which definitely were *not* made for walking, would have been ill advised even if she hadn't been pregnant, but in her state they were especially disconcerting. They may have been trendy that week, but a one-week trend does not good fashion make.

While go-gos are pretty obvious no-nos, there are plenty of other styles that should be avoided as well. Shoes are not like Mount Everest—you can't climb onto them just because they are there. There are way too many universally unflattering shoes on the market today that can trip you up—sometimes literally. Although shoe styles, like clothing styles, change from season to season, the following guidelines should keep you out of hazardous territory and shepherd you safely into the land of Camouflage Chic.

BEWARE OF THE FOLLOWING STYLES

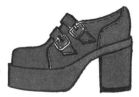

Square toes and chunky heels: Now, I know clunky, chunky, square, heavy shoes have been all the rage, but it's a given that a few seasons down the road fashion historians will dismiss them with a derisive wave of their well-manicured hands (if they haven't already). Elegant and graceful they are not. **Heavy, chunky shoes make your legs look heavy**

and shorten the whole body—unless you've got exceptionally skinny legs, in which case your legs end up looking like toothpicks. Neither scenario is especially appealing.

This doesn't mean you have to trade in your comfortable walking shoes for pointy-toed stilettos. If you like the solid feeling of chunky heels, try to find slightly modified ones that are somewhat tapered and more refined but that still give you the *feel* you want. But the broad square toes have to go. We can't have you looking as though you stubbed your entire foot.

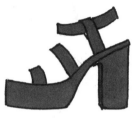

Stilettos: If you have **heavyish legs** you can get in trouble with ultra-pointy-toed stiletto heels and other ultradelicate styles. The contrast in proportion can actually make your legs look heavier. Even slingbacks are risky if your heel is the least bit pudgy. **Your best bets are styles that are neither too delicate nor too clunky.**

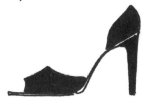

The fact is, stiletto heels are a questionable style for most everybody, regardless of leg shape. True, they elongate the leg and make for terrific *Vogue* pictures—where would Helmut Newton be without them?—but you have to wonder exactly where they fit in the context of an average woman's life. They're inappropriate for the office, debilitating on public transportation, crippling on the streets, laughable for recreation, incapacitating on errands, and suicidal when dealing with kids. Let's face it, stilettos are suited only for limousine-chauffeured dressy evenings or, if one is to believe Jerry Springer and *Cosmo,* underdressed evenings in one's boudoir.

Moreover, according to foot specialists, super-high heels thrust all your weight forward, which puts a huge amount of stress on the balls of your feet and the big toe joints and can cause all sorts of problems including bunions, hammertoes, calluses, shin splints, corns, muscle spasms, and faulty alignment. So if you must wear stilettos, at least do so in moderation, and wear them only a few hours a day. It would really be a shame in this day and age to ruin your feet in the name of fashion. Most experts agree that a 2¼-inch heel is about as high as you should go on an everyday basis. If you feel you need a bit more height proportionately, think about getting a little extra lift from a thickish sole or mini-platform.

Ultraflat flats: Since I'm totally miserable when my feet are not 100 percent comfortable, I wear flats most of the time. I love the mobility. But there are flats and there are *flats.* **Shoes with even as little as a one-inch heel, although technically flats, will give you a much longer, leaner line than a shoe that is** *totally* **flat on the bottom.** This is especially true in trousers—something to keep in mind when you buy casual shoes like loafers and skimmers. You can also get extra height, while still maintaining the comfort level, in shoes with a nice double-thick rubber sole. These days, even first-class shoe companies make wonderful casual/dressy slip-ons with thick rubber bottoms. Styles like classic sneakers and stretchy aqua-sock type shoes are incredibly comfortable, but unfortunately will *not* make you look any slimmer or taller. They are, however, wonderful to have around for those days when you're taking a fashion time-out.

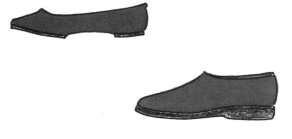

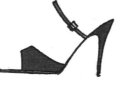

If the feet are uncomfortable, the mind is uncomfortable.

—DONALD J. PLINER, shoe designer

Manolos are always comfortable, and Guccis are gorgeous, but I probably wear Pumas and my Ugg boots more than anything else. I'm a person who ends up carrying my shoes.

—SHARON STONE, actress

Straps across the instep or around the ankles: Strappy shoes are iffy styles for anyone with less than model-perfect legs. T-straps are the worst. **The wider and darker the straps, the greater the risk.** Reason: The straps interrupt the vertical line of the leg, making the leg look shorter, the ankle wider, and the calf more noticeable. The chunky-heeled nouveau Mary Janes that were in vogue for a few minutes were universally unflattering. And to make matters worse, the style didn't really go with anything. They were an anomaly with chic suits, too heavy for little dresses, and pointless with pants.

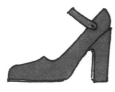

There are, on the other hand, some incredibly slim and sexy evening shoes and sandals with straps that fall across the instep. Some of those can actually look quite good, since the straps are *very narrow,* and your leg shape becomes a nonissue anyway when you're wearing long evening dresses or pants.

As for styles with straps that not only fall across the instep, but wrap around the ankles or creep up the leg, go for it if long, gorgeous gams are one of your major assets—they *will* draw attention to your lovely legs. But please give them a miss if your legs are short or heavyish. In that case, go for simple pumps or sandals that are cut relatively low in the front. *Shoes with streamlined fronts will always make your leg look longer and slimmer.*

MISSED MATCHES—WEARING THE RIGHT SHOES WITH THE WRONG OUTFITS

You've probably heard that bad food combining can give you indigestion. Well, so can bad shoe/outfit combining—metaphorically speaking, of course. It's a sort of aesthetic indigestion. Pumps and Bermuda shorts, for instance, can invite instantaneous heartburn. Stilettos with jeans are more of a squeamishness thing. *Shoes should connect organically with your outfit.* Sexy strappy sandals are lovely with a bare evening dress, ballet slippers are perfect with a long, flowing skirt, sophisticated pumps are naturals with a chic suit, loafers terrific with slacks and a blazer, boots great with jeans, sneakers with sweats, etc.

If you're just oozing personal style and have the personality and clout to carry it off—being famous, or at least involved in the arts, helps—you could go totally against type by wearing the opposite kind of footwear from what is expected. This is the **antishoe approach,** where you totally ignore all tenets of proportion and good taste and just let 'er rip—pairing Dr. Martens, say, with an evening dress or motorcycle boots with a micro-mini. In fact, *W (Women's Wear Daily's* monthly magazine), in the January 1998 issue, paired everything from a Chanel suit to a lovely calf-length Armani beaded

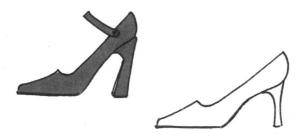

dress with Surplus Doursoux boots. The label may *sound* fancy, but they *look* like serious kick-ass army boots. The seventeen-year-old models looked *très courantes*, but would you?

> *I love wearing things that don't quite fit to-*
> *gether—like an ascot or a tie with really inap-*
> *propriate shoes. I think my shoes and jewelry*
> *look like they belong in Miami.*
>
> —TÉA LEONI, actress

That kind of flagrant fashion rebellion is about making a personal statement and flashing attitude. That's why fashion designers do it in their collections—to make a statement, not necessarily to sell a look. It provides a certain couture tension and makes for great fashion photos. It's a style that will be noticed and commented on—both negatively and positively. It's good press. Us normal folk, however, are probably better off toeing the company line and sticking to tried and true pairings. After all, **heavy shoes add weight to the whole outfit—and to you.** Anyway, you have to ask yourself, would Audrey Hepburn have worn combat boots with her Givenchys?

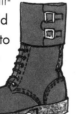

Too much shoe: When you're wearing skirts or dresses, **shoes with high horizontal vamps (the vamp is the part of the shoe that goes across the top of your foot) will make your leg look heavier.** Shoes with V-shaped vamps, or styles that scoop low, will lengthen the leg.

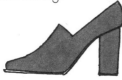

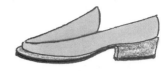

To make big feet (size nine and up) smaller, make sure your shoes are cut *to the foot*—that is, **without an extended sole** showing around the edges. If you've got skinny ankles, look for shallow shoes and try slingbacks. **Too much shoe on skinny legs produces ze look of ze toothpick.**

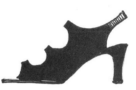

Squirrelly openings: Open-toed shoes and sandals can be winners, **but make sure the toe opening is the right shape for your feet.** If the opening is *too small,* your toe can look like the nose of a little baby rodent trying to get out of a cage. If it's *too big,* some of your other toes might look deformed as they're mashed together in the opening. Neither look is particularly fetching.

Iffy color balance—not a matter of black and white: For starters, *white pumps have to go!* I've seen women wear them with everything under the sun, from dark stockings and velvet dresses to Bermuda shorts and culottes. All I can say is, white pumps border on the offensive. Aside from the fact that they make feet look bigger and bring attention to heavy ankles, white pumps, for some mysterious reason, tend to look cheap and tacky no matter how much they cost. (There may be exceptions, but if so, I haven't seen them.) Even if your outfit has white in it, you're usually better off with another color. The only time white shoes work is in fun, casual styles like canvas skimmers, dance shoes, espadrilles, ballet shoes, and white bucks. Even white sandals are acceptable, because there's more foot and less shoe there—just a few straps. But white pumps? NO. When your inner fashion consultant is counseling white pumps, reach instead for bone, taupe, light tan, or even a subtle metallic like bronze, copper, or pewter.

As for black: everybody needs basic black shoes in their wardrobe, but that doesn't mean black shoes go with *everything.* They often look too heavy with light- to midtoned outfits—*especially pastels*—unless there's some black accent on top to balance the whole deal. So if you don't have shoes that match *exactly*—à la Imelda Marcos (where is *she* now?)—try midtoned neutrals. Good choices: bronze and copper with warm colors, and gray tones, dulled silver, or pewter with cooler colors. **In general, your shoe should be darker, not lighter, than your outfit.**

Platform sandals: These shoes are classics as far as I'm concerned—well, *trendy* classics, anyway. I admit that's a bit of an oxymoron, but here's the way I figure it: Platforms have been in and out of fashion for at least five centuries and are at least semiutilitarian. Although with our omnipresent paved streets (in the Western world anyway) we don't need platforms to keep us up out of the mud and dirt anymore, they are helpful in the kitchen when you're reaching for the balsamic vinegar on the top shelf. So if you love 'em, wear 'em. But please note: *Worn with short skirts or shorts, they will make heavy legs look heavier and skinny legs look skinnier.* Proportionately, they really look right only with pants or long skirts, and even then they may give you more of a trendy edge than you're looking for. Essentially, they're a fun young look that requires good balance to wear. Not recommended for puddle hopping or fence leaping.

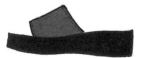

A FEW QUICK TIPS AND RECAPS

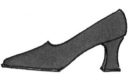

- Slim heel shapes will make you look taller and more graceful than chunky ones.

- A good general rule for short skirts: the shorter the skirt, the lower the heel. A skirt hemmed just above or below the knee, for example, can take a higher heel than a supermini (unless you're Mariah Carey). Long skirts, with the exception of formal wear, usually look best with flatter shoes or boots.

- The flatter your shoe, the more narrow your pants can be.

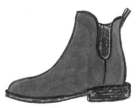

- Keeping shoes the same tone as your hose will lengthen the leg.

- Shoes with tapered toes will make the foot look longer and narrower.

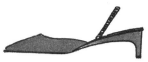

- Low vamps help lengthen the leg; high vamps shorten the leg. Low-cut pumps or low-cut slingbacks, with low to medium narrowish heels, are very flattering designs for most women.

- Lightweight textures such as silks and rayons call for a relatively light and graceful shoe. Heavier textures, such as tweeds (if you dare), call for a heavier shoe, such as sturdy English walking shoes or fine leather boots.

- A general rule of thumb for dressy shoes: The less shoe, the better the leg will look.

- When it comes to shoes, *quality* counts. Get the best you can afford.

> *Shoes are more important than suits and dresses. Buy one pair of good shoes instead of three pairs of bad quality.*
>
> —Marlene Dietrich, actress

ONE LAST THING

Shoes have more attitude than almost any other accessory. They affect not only the way you look but how you feel and move. So make sure your shoes not only are flattering but also *allow you to move with grace and ease.* Also consider if they are conveying the message you want them to. If you want

to proclaim yourself competent and brainy, sexy stilettos are probably not the way to go.

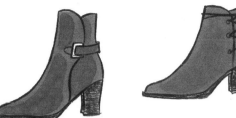

> *To keep a long skirt looking cool and boyish, it needs heavier boots or flats to get the right attitude. With heels it's elegant, formal, evening.*
>
> —Marc Jacobs, designer

HOSIERY

The kind of panty hose you choose can also move the big needle on our friendly girth meter and impact your entire look—both positively and negatively.

On the **positive side** are the three magic C-words of today's super-hose: *control, contouring,* and *compression.* Top-quality control panty hose can be every bit as effective as shapewear—and these days, they're actually quite comfy (see Rule 8 for recommendations).

PANTY HOSE DON'TS

On the negative side, the wrong panty hose can wreak sartorial havoc—and I'm not

When buying nude panty hose, test the color against your inner forearm rather than the back of your hand, which is generally darker than your legs.

even counting runs and baggy knees. Let's start with color.

- **No white panty hose!** If you have a theory about why so many women wear white hosiery, I would love to hear it. I've been pondering this one for years, and I just don't get it. **White panty hose bring attention to heavy legs and make them look bigger.** And on slim to normal legs they're just rather distasteful. Who would want white legs? As my friend Ronnie, an ex-model and un-official anti–white hose lobbyer, says, "Most people's skin turns that ashy stocking white just before it turns green and they die."

     Essentially all white hosiery should be banished from your wardrobe forever, unless you are in the medical profession. Nurses wear it because it makes their legs look germ free and sterile, which, I'm guessing, is probably not the image you're after.

- **No patterned panty hose.** The fact is, patterned panty hose are not particularly flattering. They draw unwanted attention to short or heavy legs and detract from the slim line of long slender ones. Even if the pattern is subdued, the leg can end up looking unnatural at best and diseased at worst. Vertical striped hose, which you might *think* would make your legs look longer, could actually do the opposite if you have heavy legs. Why? Because the vertical lines will curve over your calves and thighs, so instead of having stripes on your leg, you'll have a bunch of little curved lines.

- **No novelty panty hose.** This category includes *seamed stockings*, a dubious paean to the thirties; *cutesy designs*, like hose with little plastic daisies running up the back; and *black fishnet stockings*, which, need I say, are totally out of the question even at Halloween. Novelty hose are not chic and have high fat potential. Here's what happens with fishnets, for instance (I'm visualizing an old *Vanity Fair* cover photo of Barbra Streisand here as I speak): The spaces in the netting stay small and dark over the skinniest parts of your leg and spread out and lighten over the larger parts, which, of course, makes the larger parts look even larger. Then because of the contrast in color and more obvious pattern created, the eye is immediately drawn to the larger area. You might just as well wear a little neon Post-it on your thighs saying, "Hey! Looky here!"

- **Bright-colored opaque hose won't do anybody any good either.** If you pair them with a different-colored outfit, the silhouette will be broken and you will not look as long and lanky as you might otherwise. And if you wear bright opaque hose in the same color as your outfit, you could end up looking like a leprechaun (in the case of green), or Mrs. Claus (in the case of red).

A GOOD GENERAL RULE

The sportier the shoe, the more opaque the hose can be. The dressier the shoe, the sheerer the stocking should be.

I like clothes that don't clash with your personality or feel put on.

—NICOLE KIDMAN, actress

PANTY HOSE DO'S

• Nude or a shade a little darker than your skin is a perennial best bet. **Sheer black and dark gray stockings** are always quite flattering with dark skirts and very slimming to heavy legs. Just one thing to watch out for: *They must fit well,* so that the color is equally distributed on the leg and no unsightly dark dirtlike streaks appear in the crease behind the knee.

• Dark opaque hose are great in winter—again very slimming to the leg—especially when the color matches your skirt and shoes. Opaque hose, though, make for a sporty look and call for sporty shoes.

TWO LAST WARNINGS

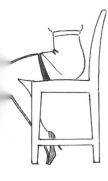

First, as I've mentioned before, *if you wear short skirts, forget about panty hose styles where the reinforced darker panty part starts on the upper thigh.* With short skirts, your panty hose should always be sheer up to the waist. I was at a meeting with a young executive last year, and when she crossed her legs I could see that un-attractive division line on her thigh. Sheer with short is the only way to go.

And finally, ***don't wear reinforced toes with sandals,*** okay? I know *you* don't do it, but I've seen it done, and it's not a good look. Sheer, sheer, sheer! In fact, why wear hose with sandals at all? You can of course, if you want to, but you don't have to. Sandals are designed to be worn on their own in warm weather. In very casual situations, why not wear socks with your sandals if your tootsies get cold? At least there's a little humor there—a sort of European tourist look that some designer will probably pick up on any day now.

BELTS

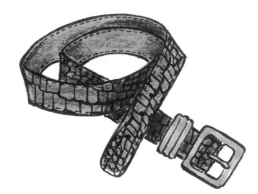

More often than not, belts add pounds.

—LEEZA GIBBONS, talk-show host

Belts can come in very handy for adding polish or shifting the proportion of an outfit, but whether *you* should wear them depends on your individual body shape. Most of us can wear belts—it's just a matter of what color, what width, and how we wear them.

A few guidelines:

- Never wear tight belts. A tightly cinched belt can make *anybody* look pudgy. As the belt cinches in the waist, it pushes all the flesh on the waist over and under the belt, so you get bulges on your hips and lower midriff. If you have to struggle to get that belt hooked in the first hole, it's time for the next size.

- Avoid contrasting colored belts. They will just create a horizontal line across your middle, shortening and widening your silhouette.

- Most women, with the exception of tall, thin ones, should steer clear of wide belts. Narrow belts work well with most body types. The heavier, bustier, shorter, or smaller you are, the narrower your belt should be.

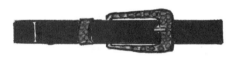

- If you're long-waisted you can wear belts a little wider, but don't overdo it, or it could accentuate short legs.

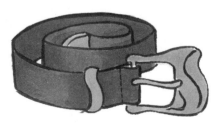

- When there is any kind of color contrast between top and bottom, long-waisted women should match their belt color to their skirt or pants to elongate the leg. Short-waisted women should match their belt to their top to elongate the torso.

- Also for short-waisted women: When belting dresses or tunics, wear belts slung low or loosely buckled, so that they V slightly in the front. When tucking tops in pants or skirts, blouse them a bit over the belt, rather than pulling them taut—a good idea for most everybody.

- Make sure the belt suits the outfit. *Just because there are belt loops, it doesn't mean that you have to wear a belt.* In fact, it's often to your advantage to remove the belt loops altogether, so that you always have the option of either going beltless or moving the belt to a more flattering position. (Since I'm short-waisted, I *always* remove belt loops on pants, so that I can *lower* my belts to *lengthen* my torso. It also works like a charm on coats and jackets.)

- Think twice about belting jackets. It almost always creates excess bulk. As a stylish friend of mine says, "I've never seen a belted jacket that wouldn't look better unbelted." And I have to agree.

- If a garment comes with a belt—especially the tacky faux leather kind—either replace it with a quality belt or eliminate it altogether.

- If you have a thick waist or midriff, you can still wear a belt—just cover up the sides of the belt with an open jacket, vest, or cardigan. The full breadth of your waist will then be hidden, the horizontal line will be shortened, and you'll still reap the style rewards.

JEWELRY

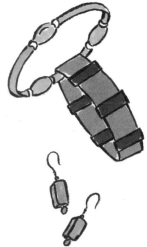

> *I don't think that tons of jewelry is ever advisable.*
>
> —ISAAC MIZRAHI, **designer**

In general, jewelry is really more about adornment, individualizing your look, and having fun with fashion than it is about camouflaging. But, in fact, most jewelry also serves as a diversionary tactic by distracting the eye from trouble spots and redirecting it to more advantageous positions. That said, some styles are definitely more advisable than others. A few specifics to consider:

• Long necklaces—strands of beads, gold, silver, or pearls—are great for creating flattering vertical lines. Try multiples of varying longish lengths. On the other hand, long strands are *not* a great idea for big-busted women, since the necklaces cascade over the bosom and are left hanging in midair. A necklace that ends above the bust is a better bet in that case.

• Bulky chokers are iffy for most everyone, since they create a horizontal line across the neck, visually separating it from the torso. They're espe-

cially lethal for short-waisted busty women, who need all the neck length they can get. **The best idea is to keep chokers on the narrow and/or flat side.**

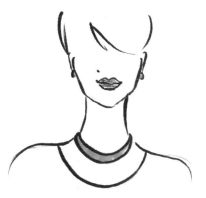

• Heavy women should avoid chunky, bulky beads and pendants and opt for styles that lie flat.

• Keep jewelry scaled to your size—not too large for small women or too small for big women. If a pin is too insignificant to stand alone, try wearing two or three together. Same for bracelets and rings. Multiples will always be fashionable.

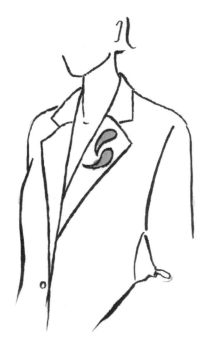

- Earrings should suit your face, style, and shape. Big, bold earrings will overpower most small faces. Strong faces call for substantial earrings. Big round earrings will make a round face look rounder.

- Drop earrings can help elongate and make you look taller, but they must be in proportion to the face and work with your hair length. If they're too long or too big, they can drag you down. Contrary to what you might think, ultralong dangling earrings will *not* help lengthen a short neck; they will, in fact, draw attention to it. Don't let dangles fall below the jawline.

HATS

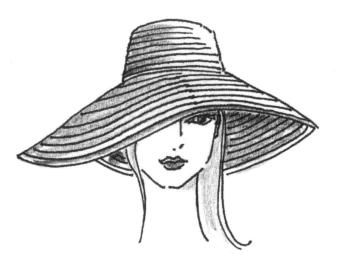

> *Hats divide generally into three classes: offensive hats, defensive hats, and shrapnel.*
>
> —KATHARINE WHITEHORN, British journalist

Unless you're a member of the royal family, chances are you're not much of a hat wearer—except perhaps for winter warmers and the occasional beret or baseball cap. Hats, alas, are becoming a bit of an anachronism for the modern working woman. Should you, however, ever have the occasion to hit the chapeau trail, here are a few quick tips:

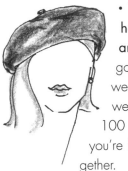

- **There should be genuine harmony between your hat and your personality.** To look good in them, you have to wear hats as naturally as if you were born in them. If you're not 100 percent comfortable in them, you're better off avoiding them altogether.

- **Hat shape must be totally complementary to your body and face shape.** Small women disappear under ultra-wide-brimmed hats. Large women look silly with pillboxes perched on their heads.

- Watch out for any big shapes that will make your neck disappear when seen from behind. Seeing the neck is essential for maximum elongation.

- Large crowns on hats add inches, but they usually look pretty ridiculous, since they throw all proportions out of whack. It's not worth the trade-off.

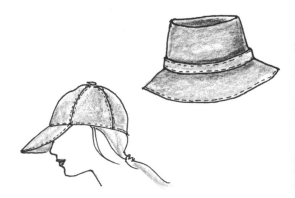

BAGS

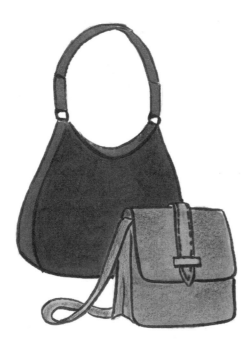

Bags, of course, should fit your lifestyle, blend nicely with your basic neutral wardrobe, and be stylish enough to take anywhere with confidence. They should also be compatible with your clothes, personality, and body type. The most important thing about bags from the *Does This Make Me Look Fat?* point of view is that they are **proportion and balance appropriate.** So keep the following in mind:

• Size contrasts can create problems, since they leave too much room for comparison. An oversized bag will make a short woman look shorter, while an undersized one will make a large women look larger.

• Be careful that straps on shoulder bags are not too long. A bag that hangs too low will also make you look shorter, because it will bring the eye down. Many bags are designed with long straps, so that you have the option of slinging the bag across your body from one shoulder to the opposite hip—which is fine *if* you wear it that way. But if you don't, what's the point? In that case, take your bags to a shoe repair shop and have them either shorten the long straps permanently or render them adjustable.

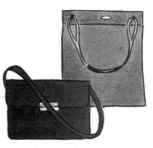

• A broad wide bag worn around the hip area will bring attention to the hips as well as create a dreaded horizontal line. Shapes that are a bit longer than wider are generally better (unless they are quite small).

- Softer bags with slightly rounded edges are generally more flattering than stiff ones with sharp angles, since they're a more natural shape.

- Bags that are too soft and floppy, or too rounded, are not recommended for heavy women, since they can almost appear to be part of the body.

- Carrying a heavy bag on your shoulder over the years can actually make one shoulder lower than other, throwing you out of balance for years to come.

HAIR

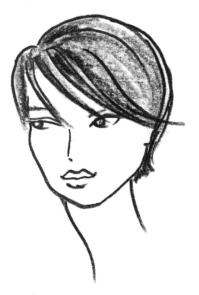

Hair shouldn't look like it's trying too hard. It's tacky.

—FREDERIC FEKKAI, hair guru

As your **ultimate accessory,** hair can be your shining glory or your horror story. It is, after all, always right up there on top of your head for the entire world to see every minute of every day. It's not as if

you can cover it up with the perfect jacket. Which explains, of course, why we all freak out on bad hair days.

In this context, though, a bad hair day is more than just how your hair is behaving on any given day. **Here, it's the effect of your hair's shape, dimension, and length on your overall proportion that counts.** While hair can't make you look fat per se, it can change your face shape, influence how tall or short you look, and strongly impact your overall proportion and balance. If you've got the wrong coif, you could be having a bad hair year—or, worse, a bad hair life without even knowing it. Too awful to contemplate, really.

People get real comfortable with their features. Nobody gets comfortable with their hair. Hair trauma. It's the universal thing.

—JAMIE LEE CURTIS, actress

A perfect coif is one that is totally compatible with your personality, lifestyle, hair texture, facial features, and—most important for our purposes—**your body type and face shape.** The best hairstylists take all those factors into consideration before they start clipping. The worst ones don't. They're more likely to give you a version of *their* favorite cut with little regard for the whole you. So if you don't already have a brilliant hairstylist, you need to get one—one who not only cuts superbly but who also has excellent taste. Do some serious research to find the best in your area—pay more if you have to. Even if you can't afford the maestro for each individual trim, just go a few times till you settle on the perfect style. Then go to someone less costly who can follow the cut—perhaps a recommended stylist in the same salon.

I don't mean to minimize the quest—finding a talented hairstylist can be tedious. *But you must prevail.* A woman in search of a good cut needs determination and fortitude. You might even have to suffer a few choppy cuts before you find a truly talented stylist. But trust me, if you're persistent he will come. I was totally traumatized when I moved from Los Angeles to Nashville and had to leave my beloved Cristophe—a genius cutter if there ever was one. I was sure I was going to be in hair hell for the rest of my life. As it turned out, I had to suffer only one atrocious haircut (and subsequent trauma) before I happened upon Jean-Charles—another genius cutter! Actually, the poor man sat next to me on a plane and had to listen to me whine about my previous atrocious cut all the way from New York to Nashville. He totally understood, though . . . and I knew I had my man. So good hairstylists are out there (and they're often French, I might add). You just have to find them. Keep your eyes peeled for women with great cuts who have hair texture similar to yours. When you spot one, diplomatically approach and ask her who cuts her hair. Most of the time she'll be flattered and happy to share her

source. If she knocks you flat, you'll make so much money on the lawsuit you'll be able to have your own hairstylist on staff. It's a win-win situation.

Meanwhile, until the fateful day when you cross paths with your very own genius superstylist, here are some general guidelines to keep in mind:

- **Head size counts** when considering balanced proportions. Since there's no way to change the actual size or shape of your head—with all your brains intact, anyway—you have to count on your hairstyle to keep your head size in proportion to the rest of your body. All things considered, it's **better to err on the small side than the large,** since big hair is totally passé and a small-ish head will make you look a bit taller and more slender.

- **Your hairstyle should be consistent with your clothing style.** Tailored classic clothing calls for a trim classic hairdo. A trendier overall image can handle a trendier do.

- **Don't get stuck in an era.** Just because your long, straight, glossy hair won you praise and adoration in the seventies doesn't mean you have to wear it that way for the rest of your life. If you are like the rest of us, your lovely face subtly changes as you age, and your hairdo should follow suit. A style that is flattering on an eighteen-year-old face may only accentuate new lines on someone older.

- **Small women:** Short is almost always the best length. Big-volume hair tends to overpower and look silly. Long hair tends to drag you down. Short, heavy women usually need a little volume lest they look like pea heads (although there are rare exceptions like my friend Gayle, who has parlayed her ultrashort cropped do into a wonderfully unique personal style).

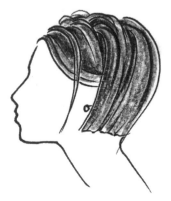

- **Big women:** Heavier women may need more volume to balance their figure, but hair should be on the short side and kept off the neck. Very long hair tends to flatten down on the scalp and only makes you seem shorter and wider. Plus, you'd lose the elongating line of the neck and end up all shoulders and head from the back. Women with full faces should try some hair close to the sides of the face.

- Hair that **caps the head** gives the illusion of shortness.

- **An asymmetrical style** can make you look taller as it brings the eye upward at an angle. So hair pulled to one side with a comb or barrette, or cut longer on one side, will contribute *imaginary* inches.

- **Naturally curly hair** will give you an *actual* inch or two on top—especially if it's longer there. Just watch out that you don't wind up with "big hair."

- Hairstyles that **show the neck** are good for most women because they create an elongating line. This is especially important for women with short necks, who should *always* wear hair above their shoulders—close to the head and above the ears is best.

- **Upsweeps** that naturally show the neck have the same lengthening effect as short hair—but keep them simple. If do's are too intricate, you can end up looking top-heavy—think Las Vegas showgirl. Also, keep knots and chignons relatively high up on the back of the head. Too low, or centered in back, creates a horizontal in profile.

- Sixties-style **long, straight, center-parted hair** pulls the face and the body down. Leave it to the Mod Squad.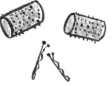

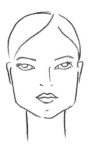

The key in going from long to short is to be cautious. You can always go further if you like.

—JOHN SAHAG, hair superstylist

FACE SHAPE GUIDELINES

Note: These are *guidelines* only. Because of the myriad other factors—such as facial features, personal style, personality, lifestyle, stature, etc.—it's impossible to choose your hairstyle by face shape alone. Plus, because face shapes are subtle, we often misjudge our own. So use the following tips as a starting point, then confer with your hairstylist. With that in mind . . .

- *Round face:* The idea here is to elongate the face, rather than adding more roundness or width. So try the following: More volume on top, less on the sides. Upswept styles. Side parts that run at a diagonal to the crown. Side, not center, parts. Avoid blunt cuts in back of the neck. Try wispy bangs or none at all. Full bangs will shorten the face.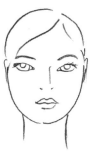

- *Square face:* An illusion of softness and some height is needed to offset the angular width and soften the jawline. To accomplish that, try more volume on top than on the sides, chin-length subtly layered cuts, asymmetrical styles, and wispy bangs. Avoid dead straight bangs and blunt cuts at the neck. Also, try pulling your hair back into a classic ponytail—always a winner.

- *Oblong face:* Bangs are great. So are layered cuts that add softness to the sides of your face and a bit of volume. Avoid long straight styles, center parts, and unnecessary height.

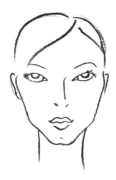

- *Heart-shaped face:* The idea here is to add more width at the jawline to balance the forehead. So try soft bangs, styles that softly cover the ears, fullness at the nape of the neck, and blunt cuts. Avoid hair that's too flat or too high.

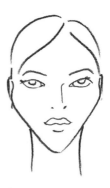

- *Triangular face:* Try styles with fullness at your jawline and over the cheekbones. Fullness low at the back of the neck will help balance your small chin. Upswept styles can work, as can asymmetrical or soft light bangs, waves, or curls that direct the eye up and out at the eyeline and above.

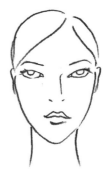

- *Oval face:* Theoretically, all styles and all lengths will work since an oval face is already well balanced. Your choices are wide open!

Whatever you put on your body, or do to your hair, or do to your face should be some sort of extension of yourself, not some trend that someone wants you to follow. The simpler, the better.

—MEG RYAN, actress

RULE 10

USE DIVERSIONARY TACTICS TO DIRECT ATTENTION TO YOUR FACE

The major principle behind this rule is pretty simple: *You won't look fat if nobody is looking at your alleged fat parts.* So the ploy is to simply divert attention away from said alleged fat parts and direct it toward your face. True, you could—and should—draw attention to your other good points, say a great pair of legs or beautiful shoulders, or gorgeous toned arms. But first and foremost is **the face—your center of communication.** That's where your true inner beauty and intelligence shine through; where your wit and charm express themselves; where your uniqueness and soul live. There is no woman who won't benefit from this strategy.

There are a number of ways to lead the eye to the face. We've already touched on a few of them: a splash of contrasting color around the neck; jewelry; and elongating necklines like V necks. Elegant negative space is another. And scarves are probably best of all.

Negative Space

In fashion, **negative space** is usually created when bare skin is surrounded by material. The shape of the material defines the negative space. Bare skin that shows though cutout sections of certain gowns, for instance, is negative space, as is the bare skin that shows around certain necklines. These are the negative spaces that concern us here—the ones formed by necklines (the other kind we can do without). Since the shape of the negative space is formed by the shape of the positive space (i.e., the neckline of your garment), you want to choose your

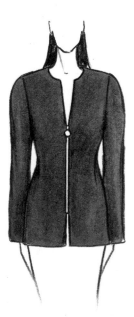

necklines very carefully. The more attractive the shape of the neckline, the better the shape of the negative space and the more effective it is at directing attention up toward your face. If all this sounds a little technical, just have a look at the following illustrations, and you'll see exactly what I mean.

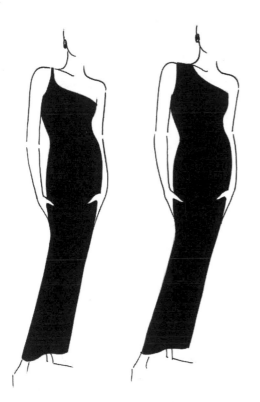

While the difference is subtle, the neckline on the left creates a more flattering negative space than the one on the right.

Scarves

Scarves are a bit like jewelry—a personal touch, a caprice, a vice.

—GIORGIO ARMANI, designer

Scarves are unbeatable when it comes to redirecting attention to your face. Plus, as they draw attention upward, they can also actually help elongate the body and easily turn an ordinary outfit into something extraordinary. That, in my book, qualifies **scarves as the number one Camouflage Chic accessory.**

While solid-colored, interestingly textured scarves in tones or values close to your outfit can be wonderfully sophisticated—picture a deep emerald with a midnight blue, or midnight blue with black—print scarves are a natural. With scarves you can add all the prints, drama, and contrasting colors you want with impunity. Finally! **Here color and fun prints get a chance to do what they do best—attract attention—only this time, just where you want it.**

Scarves come in two basic shapes, square and oblong, and a variety of sizes. Large squares are terrific when worn as shawls, but aren't as elongating as oblongs when tied or draped. They're also a little trickier to tie and a little bulky when wrapped around the neck. Small squares aren't all that flattering either. When they're tied at the neck, bandana style, they shorten a short neck and usually look a bit styled and affected on a long neck. When they're tucked into jacket breast pockets, they tend to break the clean silhouette of the design. They are, alas, rather useless.

So for my money, oblongs are the way to go. They're very easy to tie and drape, are seldom bulky, reinforce vertical lines, and are extremely versatile. There's also a certain insouciant, unstud-

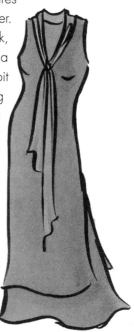

ied look about them that makes them very easy to integrate naturally into your wardrobe—and with scarves, the more effortless they look, the better.

As for fabrics, **I strongly recommend going for top quality**—silks, chiffon, charmeuse, crêpe de chine, and velvet. Think about your wardrobe, and consider the kind of clothing you'll be pairing with your scarves. Lighter-weight garments call for lighter-weight scarves. A four-ply silk scarf or a rich silk charmeuse, for instance, might prove too heavy for a crêpe jacket but could be perfect with one in light wool gabardine. Likewise, feathery chiffon might look unbalanced with a wool jacket but be perfect with summer linen.

Good scarves can be expensive, but the perfect scarf—one that is ideally suited to you and your style—is a worthwhile fashion investment. Think of it as cloth jewelry. It will elevate and upgrade any outfit you wear, and since it will never go out of style, you'll be able to wear it for years and years. I can't tell you the number of times my favorite oblong hand-printed silk scarf has added zip to my various basic black outfits. I practically had a coronary arrest the day I shelled out $150 for that scarf—but in the long run it was worth every penny. It has already paid for itself in triple when I consider how many times it's pulled me out of major fashion predicaments.

My ever-stylish sister Eda, though, is *the* major scarf maven in the family. She wears one practically every day and has a collection that I unabashedly covet. Since she's also a brilliant shopper, I asked her to share her scarf-buying secrets with us, which she happily did. Here, then, are Eda's tips from the field:

To me, a scarf is a significant investment, so I'll stand and futz with one for half an hour to make sure it's going to work for me. I throw it around my neck and try tying and knotting it several different ways to make sure it holds the way I want it to. If a scarf is too stiff or too soft, the knot won't hold well. . . . If I think I'm going to be looking at scarves, or have any notion that I'm going to be shopping that day, I try to wear a blazer, something I would naturally wear a scarf with, rather than trying to imagine it while wearing something completely different.

Also, I've always found that when I'm in a store that sells expensive scarves, there is invariably a knowledgeable salesperson there. And if they want to help you, let them. If they tie the most fabulous knot and you think you could never do it, let them show you how—which, by the way, is done with you in front of a mirror with them *behind you*, not in front of you. It's a little close contact for some people. But if you can tolerate it, it's easier to copy what they're doing. If they're facing you and tying it, you'll never get it. The better the store, the more likely you'll find someone who's going to have the patience. If they want to sell a two-hundred-dollar scarf and you say, "Gee, this looks kind of wide, how's it going to look?" they'll show you how to work with it.

Meanwhile, until you hook up with a super saleslady, here are some of my favorite ways to tie, wrap, and drape scarves. After you try these, play around and experiment on your own. You'll probably be able to come up with some of your own inventions—which you can then share with *your* saleslady.

> *You can buy black separates that aren't especially expensive, but when you put them together with a good scarf and a good pocketbook the whole outfit looks really upscale.*
>
> —EDA BARUCH, producer

Slimming ways to wear oblong scarves:

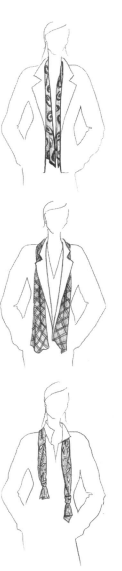

- *Hanging straight down just **inside your jacket.*** This looks best with collarless tops such as shells and V necks. The scarf not only creates vertical lines but also covers belly, bust, waist, etc.

- *Hanging over your jacket, **under the lapels.*** This is sometimes a better look if the blouse you're wearing with the jacket has a collar, or if you're wearing necklaces. The scarf will still create a nice vertical line, but you won't have too much bulk around your neck.

- *Hanging straight down over or under a jacket, but **knotted on each side.*** The knots add weight to keep the scarf hanging straight. They're also a great way to adjust the length. A one-sided knot also works. Obviously, the scarf has to be made of a relatively lightweight fabric or the knot will be too bulky.

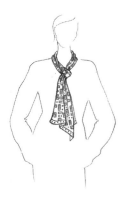

- *Hacking knot.* This one is incredibly easy. Just fold the oblong in half lengthwise, place around your neck, and slip the two ends through the center fold loop. Adjust to taste. This works like a dream with longer narrow scarves.

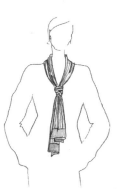

- *Slipknot.* Hang the scarf around your neck, tie a loose knot in one side, slip the other side through the knot, adjust the height of the knot to the most flattering position—which depends on where your jacket button falls, what kind of jewelry or belt you're wearing, the length of your top, collar type, etc.

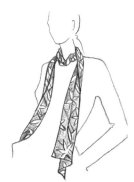

- *Neck wrap.* Wrap the scarf once around your neck and leave the ends hanging straight on both sides. Great with shells and other round-necked tops.

- *Neck wrap tie.* Tie a loose knot in the middle of the scarf, place the knot under your chin. Cross ends behind your neck and bring them back to the front. Slip the ends through the knot, going in opposite directions. Tighten knot to suit. Wear either in front or to the side.

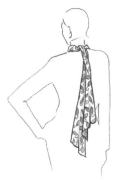

• *Wrapped around the neck and left hanging in the back East Indian style.* Very stylish with very simple outfits. Not great with jackets.

Once you start wearing scarves, there's a good chance you'll get hooked. But if you buy wisely, scarves will ultimately prove a much more worthwhile addiction than some others I could mention—like chocolate.

> *With the right earrings, bracelet, and scarf, you will always be very too-too.*
>
> —WENDY WASSERSTEIN, playwright, from *The Sisters Rosensweig*

SOME FINAL TIPS

• Wear scarves in colors that warm your skin and make it glow. Unless you are a very pale blonde, who can use taupe as one of your base colors, beiges and very pale colors could wash you out.

Camel, mustard, and pea green are also very risky colors for most skin tones.

• A printed scarf should always include some of the same colors as your outfit.

• Scarves with silver or gold thread running through them, or with beads or sequins, are fabulous evening accessories when worn with basic black. They can turn a simple black outfit into a masterpiece.

• Go for dramatic scarves, rather than neutral ones.

• Check street fairs and craft fairs for potential good deals on hand-painted silk scarves.

• Gauge widths according to your neck length. Long necks can handle wider widths. If your neck is short, look for narrower scarves or very soft wide ones, which can be folded in half widthwise before you drape or tie them.

• Heavier women generally do better with thinner scarves.

• Short women, watch that you don't wear scarves too long.

• The smaller or narrower the scarf, the smaller the pattern should be.

RULE 11

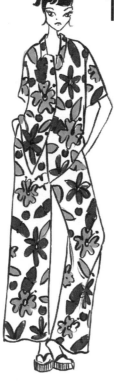

THINK SMALL

Thinking small doesn't mean being narrow-minded—lord knows we have enough of that in the world. What it means is this: Anytime you have a *design* choice (not a *size* choice)—between something large and something small, you're generally better off going for the smaller. That means smaller lapels, smaller pockets, smaller buttons, and smaller prints. The words you don't want cluttering your fashion vocabulary are ones like *broad, wide, big, flared, chunky,* etc. **One good rule of thumb: If you wouldn't like the word to describe you in general, it shouldn't describe any portion of your wardrobe, either.** We've already touched on a few of the large-size offenders: hunky shoulders, chunky jewelry, clunky shoes, big hair, and the like. But there are still some at large that need to be addressed.

No Big Prints!

I'm still a big believer in solid colors as the mainstay of a wardrobe, but it's perfectly acceptable to incorporate a few prints from time to time—just not those big loud tropical prints, unless, of course, you're at a luau. The eye gets very confused amid all those pineapples and hibiscuses. It ends up going around and around, and when it does you look bigger and bigger. Subtle prints are much easier on the eye—and your figure. Here's how to do prints:

- **Keep the pattern small and/or sparse.** Look at a potential print through squinted eyes. If it starts to blend together and look more like a texture than a print, it's a good *small print.* A good *sparse print* has just an occasional image—say, an elephant or a jug (not teddy bears, I hope)—scattered around on the fabric.

- **Keep the background dark.** This is the same principle as dark solids (see Rule 2). The background recedes, instead of advances, and you look smaller.

- **Look for prints in which the image and background are close in value.** That way you get almost the same slimming effect afforded by solids, with the additional interest of a print.

- **Prints with angles** (not angels) will be more slimming than prints with a lot of curves, swirls, and curlicues.

• **If you ever mix prints with plaids or other patterns,** keep them all in the same color family, and make sure that one print is dominant over the others.

Buttons

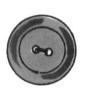

Buttons are by nature round (you'll excuse me for stating the obvious). When buttons are oversized, they are both big and round. *Big round things are not what you want on your body.* The only thing worse than oversized buttons is oversized *shiny* buttons, which, unfortunately, seem to have found favor with a lot of inexpensive and midrange clothing manufacturers. Who knows why? Big cheap shiny buttons are not only *extremely* tacky, they also limit your accessories and have fat potential, which plops them smack into the "things to avoid" category.

The best thing about buttons, though, is that they are very easy to remove or replace. **A simple button switch can completely rejuvenate a jacket or coat in a flash.** So look through your closet and see if there are any garments in there that could use a button makeover. Replace cheap faux silver and gold buttons with subtle bone ones in the same tone as the garment, and try slightly smaller ones if the garment can handle the proportion difference. **The more subtle your buttons, the better.** Also think about totally removing extraneous buttons—that is, buttons that are there merely for decoration.

Collars and Lapels

There's no real point to large wide lapels or big floppy collars as far as I'm concerned. It's a seasonal hype thing more than anything else. One season lapels and collars will be shown narrow, the next they'll be bigger and wider. But who really cares? Regardless of what's in vogue, narrower

---

T I P

Check any garments you're getting rid of for high-quality buttons. You might want to keep them as possible future replacements. Also, keep button switcheroos in mind when you're shopping in antique or secondhand shops—there might be old garments there that are worth buying just for the classy buttons. Sometimes the only thing keeping a garment from being a winner is the buttons, so off with the bad and on with the good.

lapels and smaller collars (or no lapels or collars at all) are always more slimming—and that goes for jackets, shirts, coats, and dresses.

If you're a lot narrower on top than on the bottom, you could use *slightly* wider lapels, perhaps, to help balance the discrepancy—but only slightly wider or you'll end up looking wide from top to bottom.

The problem with wide lapels is that they create horizontal lines, so they tend to make round faces look rounder and necks and torsos look shorter. Ditto for big floppy collars. So I say stick to narrower lapels and smaller collars—wait out the wide times.

Pockets

The only good big pockets are the ones you can't see. The other ones should be small or, better yet, nonexistent. The big pockets that bother me the most are the kind that are on safari jackets and the like—big square patches that are often stitched in a contrasting color thread or trimmed in some awful contrasting piping. Basically they just add bulk—and God forbid you should put anything in them.

Also, watch the placement of false pockets with rectangular flaps. You don't want flaps on your hips—especially if they're piped in a contrasting color.

RULE 12

KEEP IT SIMPLE

> To my mind, simplicity is the keynote of all true elegance.
>
> —COCO CHANEL, designer

This is the mother of all Camouflage Chic rules. I often think of it as the *sweep rule,* since it cleans up any minor offenses that may have slipped through the cracks of the other rules. Simplicity is such a timeless philosophy that if you followed no other rule but this one, you'd still be well ahead of the game. Simplicity doesn't mean boring or unadorned. It means *not overadorned.* It's the absence of the clutter and extraneous embellishment that can interfere with sleek clean lines and steal your thunder. **It's part of what Yves Saint Laurent meant when he said, "The woman should wear the clothes, the clothes should not wear the woman."** Too many frills, flounces, and flourishes, too much fuss and fancy, and your clothes will wind up wearing you. *Simplicity is the key to chic—and Camouflage Chic.*

The only exceptions to this rule are those rare women who can actually create some kind of wonderful eccentric personal style from excess and embellishment. I'm thinking specifically of the British poet Dame Edith Sitwell, who often wore cowled headpieces, gold brocade robes, and huge jet and ivory rings. With her strong Byzantine features and unusual height (six feet), she would have been an imposing figure regardless of what she wore, but her fashion choices turned her into something quite extraordinary. Now, there's no way you could call her getups simple, but the whole look worked—on her. The rest of us simply don't have the majestic presence to pull off that kind of outré individualism—or the lifestyle either, for that matter. I doubt that Dame Edith ever had to carpool.

> I loathed the way I looked [when I was young]—too exotic, and not blond. Not cute. But we see what happens to cute later on.
>
> —ANGELICA HUSTON, actress

Eccentrics and the cutting-edge avant-garde aside, most of us mere mortals would be better following in the footsteps of the more subtle women of style such as Audrey Hepburn, Katharine Hepburn, Jackie O., Slim Keith, Babe Paley, et al., who, while incredibly chic, were never overshadowed by their fashions. That said, let's discuss a few red flags.

> She was always well groomed, there was a consequential good taste in the plainness of her clothes, the blues and grays and lack of luster that made her, herself, shine so.
>
> —TRUMAN CAPOTE,
> describing Holly Golightly in *Breakfast at Tiffany's*

Ruffles

It's time to let them go. **Ruffles** are best suited for females under the age of eight—with perhaps the exception of flamenco dancers, who need them to fling around. Ruffles around necklines, or on the bottom of skirts or blouses, are obvious risks since they create horizontal lines, but even ruffles that run vertically down the front of a blouse are just a bit much, and usually tacky. They aren't chic. They're old hat and unsophisticated. You don't need them. **Plus, really, would you want to wear anything they named a potato chip after?**

Trimmings and Bindings

This category encompasses all of the extraneous ornamental edgings, borders, bands, ribbons, bows, and tassels often found on women's clothing. They're especially conspicuous on maternity frocks but can be found in every fashion subset.

Frankly, I never got the whole trimming and binding thing—especially in contrasting colors on suits. What's the point? Just a lot of superfluous lines, if you ask me. They usually confuse the eye and limit accessories. Plus, have you noticed that there are **always more trimmings on inexpensive clothing than on the good stuff?** Maybe midrange clothing manufacturers think that a little extra razzmatazz will take your mind off the questionable design and fabric of the garment. My advice: Pause, stop, and question any trimming. You don't have to eliminate it—just question it. Ask yourself, why is it there? What does it do to improve the design of the garment? How is it working for me? If you don't get satisfactory answers to those questions, then pass.

Appliqués

Appliqués are even more bothersome than extraneous trimming. For some reason, cut-rate manufacturers love appliqués. I'm a big fan of places like Target and Kmart for simple hang-out cotton V-neck sweaters and cardigans. When I find good ones I'll buy a few, wear them to death for the season, and then relegate them to the rag pile. They're low-anxiety clothing, perfect for gardening, dog washing, hiking, and grocery shopping. If they get crushed, crumbled, or spilled on, who cares? **Anyway, I can't tell you how many perfect double-ply cotton pullovers and such I've seen ruined with**

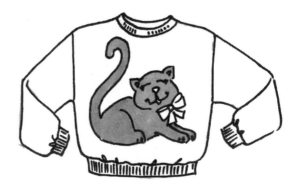

pussycat appliqués. And it's not as if it's cheaper to manufacture the garments that way. In fact, each pussycat probably costs another penny and a half. So it's beyond me. All I can tell you is that pussycats, bunnies, skunks, lightning bolts, dogs, daisies, or whatever else they tack on are not the look you're after. They won't do a thing to create a long, sleek line.

Even with inexpensive hang-out clothing, try to buy simple, slimming shapes that you can accessorize and individualize to suit your own personal style. So as you're looking through your closet or a store rack, think, Does that chambray shirt really need the embroidery on the pocket? Does that little suit really need that velvet collar? Does that belt really need all those faux silver studs? The answer is usually no.

Jewelry

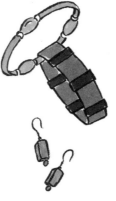

> *For a big evening, if I wear big earrings, no necklace. If I wear a necklace, no earrings or very small earrings.*
>
> —SALMA HAYEK, actress

Jewelry is a great way to dress up simple basic shapes and turn an outfit into something special. The simpler your outfit, the more jewelry you can get away with. Just remember this: **To wear a lot of jewelry well means to wear it effortlessly.** The minute it starts to look ostentatious and showy, it smacks of the arriviste. Jewelry has to look natural and blend with your personal style. If you have a penchant for overdoing it, try the old ploy of always removing one piece of jewelry before leaving the house. It still works. *Too little is always better than too much.* Little or no jewelry looks purposely minimalist. Too much just looks tacky and overdone.

If you are prone to wearing a lot of jewelry, you're always better off with multiples—that is, a grouping of the same sort of jewelry instead of a smattering of different kinds. Better to wear an armful of bracelets, a clutter of pins, a bunch of gold chains rather than one each of all of them. It's your basic gardening principle—a swath of tulips is much more effective than one tulip here and one tulip there.

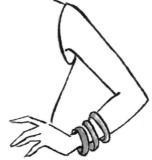

A few more gems:

- **Think balance.** If you're wearing substantial earrings, forget the necklace and add only bracelets. If you're wearing a substantial necklace, wear only the smallest stud earrings. With an armful of bracelets, forgo the necklace and add medium to small earrings. You get the idea.
- **Always decide on your jewelry in front of a full-length mirror**—it's the whole picture that counts. Nobody sees you just from the waist up unless you're a news anchor.

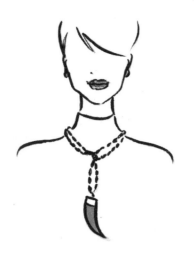

- **Play around and experiment.** Even the most fashion-savvy women try on a few different looks and combinations before they get it right. The same jewelry will look very different with different outfits.

- For more dash without too much flash, mix just a touch of silver or gold with jewelry that's in the same tones as your outfit. Almost all dark neutral colors, for instance, would look great with onyx, dark jade, fabulous woods, or varying shades of carnelian or other minerals. Then introduce some silver or gold rope for a little sparkle.

3

THE BIG FOUR—
THE MOST COMMON MISTAKES
WE WOMEN MAKE

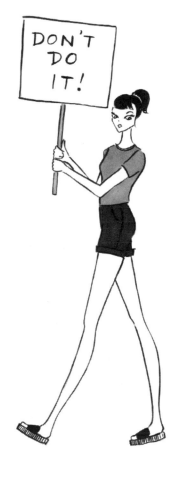

I wear what makes me feel good, not

something a designer says is current.

—HALLE BERRY, actress

The preceding twelve rules will definitely keep you on the straight and narrow, but there are still a few pitfalls lurking around that could undermine your new svelte look. **These are common universal mistakes that *everybody* makes from time to time**—so don't take them personally. Even absolutely fabulous celebrities get snagged by these traps occasionally.

In fact, across the board, celebrities make many more fashion faux pas than us plain folks, since they get invited to so many events. Each new event requires a sprightly new eye-catching getup. And every new getup presents the potential for disaster—especially if the celebrity is consciously trying to hone the cutting edge of fashion. It's simple style mathematics, really (coming soon to a junior college near you): *The more often you completely change your entire look, the higher the potential for fashion fiascoes.*

The celebrity fashion goof ratio is somewhat offset by the professional advice and assistance many of them get from top designers, stylists, and personal shoppers. But even with expert help many of them manage to make outstanding miscalculations, most of which, much to their mortification, are seized on by the international media. Luckily, *our* fashion mistakes are somewhat more regional and not usually recorded for posterity. There's something to be said for The Lives of the Not So Rich and Famous.

The marvelous thing about celebrity calamities, though, is that you can learn from them without suffering one iota of humiliation yourself. It's a painless, free education. Consider one of Paula Abdul's most photographed whoppers, for instance: vibrant blue skin-tight leather jeans, paired with a form-fitting metallic textured top with a fluffy boa-like feathered scoop neckline and cuffs, and platform stiletto leather boots. Oops, Paula didn't follow the rules! The tight shiny leather made her derriere and thighs look heavier and actually accentuated her short stature (Rule 7), and the big puffy feathers were too overwhelming for her small frame (Rules 11 and 12). There were, in all fairness, a couple of positive things about the dubious ensemble: It was monochromatic, which helped create the illusion of a bit more length (Rule 1), and the height of the heel helped the proportion some (Rule 4). But still, the outfit has to be categorized as a colossal flop. The leather and feather combo was a sartorial gamble that just didn't pay off.

While we're on the subject of feathers . . . Remember Geena Davis's much-maligned "Big Bird" Oscar dress of many years back? It was a low-cut white satin gown with black spaghetti straps and a huge poofy ruffled miniskirt that turned into a long ruffled bustle/train affair in the back. Geena wore it with black stockings and black strappy pumps. With that in mind, you have to wonder what she was thinking when she said, "I don't believe you can make a fashion mistake." Her total misses and near misses run off the charts. I recently saw an old picture of her wearing a gray plaid miniskirted suit with transparent red stockings that made her legs look piteously sunburnt. I think that qualifies as a legitimate miss, but hey, maybe that's just me.

> I believe that if your clothes wear you, it isn't modern. I'm after much more subtlety. I want the woman and her personality, her own eccentricity, and her own sense of self to come through. I'd like to hope my clothes do that for a woman.
>
> —VERA WANG, designer

Okay, moving right along . . . Now let's shift the focus away from Hollywood glitz and back to where it really matters—ourselves. I'm just guessing that fluffy azure feathers and gauzy red stockings are not some of your common pitfalls. Our biggest blunders are usually slightly less colorful and a bit more mundane—and they almost all start with general misconceptions about fashion. So let's get to it.

MISTAKE 1: FOLLOWING FADS

> Trendy is not chic, not elegant, not something that stays.
>
> —STEFANO GABBANA, designer

This is a biggie. Following fads can get you into serious trouble—even worse, the degree of severity actually increases exponentially with your age. The younger you are, the more you can get away with jumping on the latest fashion bandwagon. We expect teenagers to be into the latest, hottest thing—whether it's body glitter, tattoos, platform sandals, or Leonardo DiCaprio. They need to be accepted, part of the gang, not left out. Style over substance is the name of the game for teens, and it's perfectly acceptable—even semi-adorable.

In adults, it's less precious. Blue nail polish loses its appeal on older hands, and nobody over fifteen looks cute emulating the Spice Girls. Plus, I think it's just possible that following fads could be the result of a defective developmental link. Theoretically our twenties are a gradual mellowing-out phase, a time when it begins to dawn on us that dressing exactly like everybody else is not necessarily crucial to survival or even desirable. During our thirties our tastes become more sophisticated, creative, and individual. Easing on into our forties, our personal style peaks, and there's a natural confluence between who we are and what we wear. From fifty on we just relax and enjoy our well-earned confidence and flair.

So when a fifty-year-old woman pops up wearing the latest see-through crochet dress over a little shiny bra and bikini panties, it's not as amusing or forgivable as it might be on a twenty-one-year-old. Even if the fifty-year-old woman is in great shape, it's shaky at best. You have to ask why she's still trying so hard. What is she trying to say? In the end, it doesn't really matter. Because the message that's being delivered is decidedly déclassé. **It doesn't make sense to compete with teenagers in the fad arena.** You will never come out the winner.

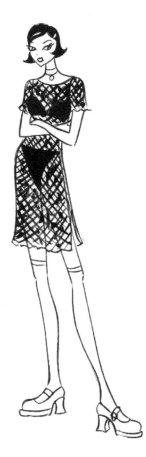

I go for classics, like Audrey Hepburn. I try to be elegant, try not to be clowny. I really hate being too hip. It makes me feel like a dog in pajamas.

—JEWEL, singer

The Difference Between Trends and Fads

That doesn't mean we should disregard *all* trends after we pass puberty. Not at all. Trends are different from fads. *Trends are general directions in mood and shape*—as in a trend toward romanticism, minimalism, or more narrow silhouettes. We're all affected somewhat by trends—although, in some cases, subconsciously. When you somehow just don't feel right in your old favorite broad-shouldered baggy jacket, you are more than likely instinctively reacting to a trend toward more fitted silhouettes. And that's perfectly legitimate. If we didn't pay attention to *general* trends we'd look as if we were stuck in a time warp, totally out of sync with everything around us. The trend in hairstyles these days, for instance, is loose and casual. You'd look very odd in a tight, controlled fifties bob.

Fads, on the other hand, are like little bleeps on the trend graph—short-term exaggerated snippets of the broad concept. A snippet of the recent narrower silhouette trend, for instance, was skintight clothing and stiletto heels—a pretty risky little look for most of us. **So keep your eye on the big picture, flow with the natural trends, and just say no to snippets that can compromise your individuality and turn you into a fashion victim instead of a style victor.**

It pains me physically to see a woman victimized, rendered pathetic by fashion.

—YVES SAINT LAURENT, designer

Exception: Every once in a blue moon, a particular fad may come along that is especially flattering or complementary to your personal style—a style that actually works *for* you instead of against you. Should one of these miracles occur in your lifetime, go for it. Hey, even stock up! If it's really *you*, you'll be able to wear it long after the blip has bleeped. I'm ecstatic every time fashion magazines mention the magic words "Asian influence," because I love mandarin collars. I'm always looking for them. So fad or no fad, when mandarin collars hit the stores, I'm there. **If a style is especially well suited to you—if you *own* that style, so to speak—then you won't look like anyone else; everyone else will look like you.**

There is also the **amusement factor exception.** Sometimes fads are just plain fun—and I'm always for anything that can provide a good chuckle. If you treat a fad with a sense of humor, you'll considerably reduce the risk of looking like a fashion victim. It's an attitude thing. A pair of lime green jelly sandals worn in summer with a soft white little sundress could be kind of amusing—sort of like a little salute to pop culture.

On the other hand, things like those schoolgirl pleated skirts that were such a rage for spring 1998 are another story. They were dowdy on everyone, and there was nothing even slightly ironic about them—except perhaps the fact that some women actually thought they would look good in them. **Truly, the only way to wear fads like that is with a touch of irreverence.** If you paired the skirt with white socks and sneakers or some other semisatirical accessory, you might not look chic, but at least you'd be indicating that you weren't taking the whole look too seriously. But really, why even bother with them in the first place?

And last, needless to say, never spend a bundle for anything that even hints of faddishness. Fads are much too short-lived to invest in heavily—that little pleated skirt fad was over before I had a chance to laugh.

> *I don't revisit anything that was ugly the first time. . . . With an outfit, what matters is if you look pretty, if it's cut well, and if the fabric's nice.*
>
> —GWYNETH PALTROW, actress

MISTAKE 2: NOT FINDING A UNIFORM

> *There's no point in trying to look like a Vogue editorial every month. The way to find your style is to try to develop a look of your own, something of you, that people can identify with you.*
>
> —CALVIN KLEIN, designer

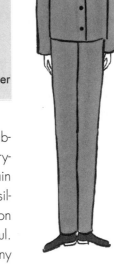

Nobody, as we've established, looks good in everything. We all have certain styles, shapes, colors, and silhouettes that look: A. great on us, B. just okay, or C. awful. Most of us own way too many of the B category—clothes that are fine, in and of themselves, but do nothing for us. They might not make us look fat exactly, but they're not sleek and slimming either. They're what I call duds.

One of the reasons they're hogging space in the closet is because we've got this thing about variety. For some reason we think we need all sorts of different styles in our wardrobes—a little of this, a little of that. But we really don't. Who says we have to look completely different every day? The truth is, we'd be *much* better off sticking to the few styles that really play up our assets and forget about all the rest—even if our wardrobes do take on a certain uniformity. What's wrong with uniformity—uniform dressing is great!

Uniform Dressing

Uniform dressing in the Camouflage Chic scheme of things simply means finding a **limited set of styles, lines, and colors that are perfectly suited to your body, personality, and lifestyle,** and making them the mainstay of your wardrobe. It means not running all over the fashion map. It's the general silhouettes, more than the actual clothes, that become your uniform—and a recognizable mark of your personal style. Katharine Hepburn's uniform was undoubtedly her turtleneck and trousers; Diana Vreeland's was her cashmere sweaters, slacks, and large pieces of exotic jewelry; and Audrey Hepburn's was slim silhouettes and unadorned simplicity. Even many of Princess Di's sheaths were similar in shape and design once she found her style.

Uniform dressing doesn't mean you'll always look the same. Your basic styles will look considerably different depending on how you wear them. And you can always add the element of surprise, fun, and interest with different accessories, textures, and innovative mixes. Uniform dressing really means that there is a common stylistic thread running throughout your wardrobe that is especially complementary to you. Think of it as "unpredictable uniformity" if that feels better.

The bottom line is that once you find what works for you—and the Rules of Camouflage Chic should definitely help you in that respect—there's just no reason to keep on wearing things that don't flatter, just for the sake of variety. If you look better in skirts than pants, then the majority of your bottoms should be skirts (if your lifestyle permits). If V necks are more flattering than scoop necks, why even have scoop necks in your closet? If long jackets suit you better than short ones, skip the short. If you look fabulous in red, why lower your wattage in camel? You get the idea. Once you start thinking in uniform terms you'll probably end up wearing more than just 20 percent of your wardrobe—as most of us do.

Naturally your uniform will take on new dimensions and evolve as fashion shifts and your tastes change. *Uniforms aren't carved in stone.* They last for an undefined period of time, ranging from a few weeks to a few years to forever. But the goal will always be the same—to be able to reach into your closet and quickly pull out something that looks absolutely fabulous on you, even with your eyes shut. You have to admit that's a lovely fantasy. And it's doable!

> *Dressing is all about signals. You can tell a whole story by the way someone puts things together. Everything is a symbol; it depends how you use it. When you wear a T-shirt with a Chanel logo, you're representing the whole idea behind it—but if you wear it with combat pants you're saying something really different.*
>
> —DESIREE MEJER, designer

MISTAKE 3: CHOOSING QUANTITY OVER QUALITY

> *Worn quality looks better than perfect junk.*
>
> —DAVID O'GRADY, artist

I know that here in America consumerism is built into our genes, and I'm not about to jinx the economy by suggesting that we have tainted DNA. So buy, buy, buy—spread the wealth—just don't do it at the expense of quality. **The truth is, you don't need more clothes, you need better clothes.** Singular excellence always triumphs over multiple mediocrity—one perfect garment is worth twenty just-passable ones. Which is why the Camouflage Chic mantra is **More is not better, better is better.**

> *You don't need a lot of clothes. Just buy very well made clothes that are simple and of very good quality.*
>
> —FERNANDO SÁNCHEZ, designer

As we've just discussed, most of us are limited by the styles we can wear well anyway. So it's not numbers that are going to bring out the best in us, it's **high-quality** clothes. Quality is a condition of excellence. In fashion, that translates to top-grade fabrics, superior workmanship, and excellent design, which, in our case, slims and trims. That's not what you usually find at low to midrange stores.

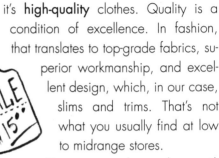

Your average low-end to moderate mass merchandise is manufactured as inexpensively as possible, designed to appeal to the most common denominator, and sized to fit most of the people most of the time. Drape, fit, silhouette, fine detailing, and elegance are not high priorities—if indeed they're considered at all. Sure, you can luck into good pieces that just happen to work occasionally—especially if you're relatively well proportioned. And those pieces are fine as filler, but it would be risky to base your entire wardrobe on them. *To look sleek and chic, you have to invest in some top-quality pieces.* How many depends strictly on the state of your finances. If money is no object, buy only the best. If budget is a consideration, you need a plan. . . .

Investment Buys

Your best bet is to buy the most important and versatile basic pieces first—a great jacket that goes with everything, the perfect skirt or pair of trousers, a flawless cashmere turtleneck or cardigan, a stunning scarf. Then slowly add more quality pieces as you find great deals and as your finances allow. If the items are high-quality, timeless classics that are flattering, slimming, and suit your style to a T, they will immediately raise the level of whatever moderately priced garments you pair with them. And even though these kinds of wardrobe staples are true **investment buys,** they don't have to cost an arm and a leg if you keep your eyes open and shop the sales.

In the long run, though, the real test of an investment buy is not how much you pay for a piece but how often you wear it and how much you enjoy it.

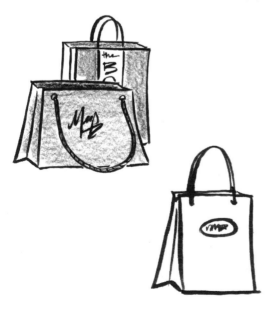

When a garment is totally flattering and a good match with your lifestyle, you'll find yourself wearing it a lot. In the end, it practically pays for itself. Say, for example, you bought a $500 jacket and wore it 150 times the first year. Your average cost per wear would be only $3.33—and that's not even factoring in bonus points for pleasure, chic, comfort, and confidence. The second year would average out at about $1.66. What a bargain! Definitely a better deal than a $100 jacket that never looks or feels quite right when you put it on.

The idea is to spend the big money where it counts—on garments that affect your silhouette and shape, not on overpriced items like designer T-shirts that have nothing special to offer except their label. I actually saw some $180 designer tank tops in the store the other day that were virtually indistinguishable from $18 mass-market ones. True, they were a lovely linen knit instead of cotton, but they looked and felt like cotton and wouldn't have much impact one way or another on your final look. It would be smarter to take the extra $162 and put it toward a fabulously chic jacket or pair of trousers—the slim and trim kind.

As your quality wardrobe slowly builds, just remember that you don't need a daring new ensemble for every day of the week. There is no longer a stigma attached to being seen in the same clothes more than once. And knowing how to mix and match to get the most out of a few pieces is a sure sign of fashion savvy. Tacky quality, on the other hand, *is* a bit of a stigma. Cheap looks cheap . . . and worse, it can actually make you look fat.

What to Look For in Top-Quality Clothes

In these days of limited expectations, even so-called quality merchandise can fall short of perfection, but if you spend a lot of money on a garment it should meet at least a good percentage of the following standards:

- Dyed-to-match zippers, completely concealed in expertly sewn plackets
- Straight seams that neither pucker nor pull (on garments *and* linings); finished edges; even stitching
- Generous seam and hem allowances
- Silk or silk taffeta lining (when lining is called for) that matches the garment, in no way interferes with its drape, and *never* shows at the hemline
- Invisible hemline stitching; hand-rolled hems on very delicate or transparent fabrics
- Matching buttons that meet straight on with buttonholes and are sewn on with stems and backed with reinforcement discs if fabric is heavy, or reinforced with a small square of matching fabric if material is delicate
- Deep, roomy pockets on trousers
- Patterns that match up at the seams, pockets, and collars
- Perfect fit (see Rule 5)

A Last Word on Labels

Most designer labels can serve as a fairly good quality gauge because top designers use better fabrics, understand the principles of fashion, and are putting their name on the line (pun intended). Labels can even indicate to some degree how a garment may fit, since designers tend to use the same fit models, which makes for some consistency in sizing. Plus, labels are a good philosophical starting point. You know from the get-go, for instance, that an Armani will be more traditional and classic than a Todd Oldham, or that a Calvin Klein will be considerably less flashy than Versace.

A particular label, however, doesn't guarantee that every garment bearing it will be a gem (even Picasso's work was not *all* museum quality) or that it will be particularly well suited to you. Designers, after all, are in business, and these days that means turning out a new collection every three months. So the creative pressure is always 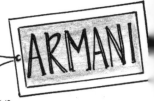 on to come up with something different and exciting. If designers did the same old thing every season—even the same *exquisite* thing—fashion editors would get bored, the designers would soon lose their cachet, and eventually they would go out of business. So they need to take chances and go out on a limb occasionally to keep things interesting—and you need to be intelligently discriminating (hence this book). Just remember, you get points for chic, not for a hot label.

MISTAKE 4: NO ORGANIZATION

We organize our kids, our households, our careers, our vacations, maybe even our husbands, so why is it we don't organize our fashion lives? We stand in front of full closets that offer us "nothing to wear." And when we do start pulling things out, some things are too big, others are too small. Or we don't have the right bra for some dresses, the right panties for some pants, the right shoes for some outfits, the right jewelry, scarves, etc., etc., etc. It's all too frustrating—and doesn't make for brilliant fashion decisions, either. We wind up settling and walking out the door in something that could, under the right circumstances, look great and maybe even slimming, but instead looks average and possibly fat. Not good. Clean up, sort out, and organize. Hedge your bets. Have the things you need to complete any outfit you own all lined up and ready to go.

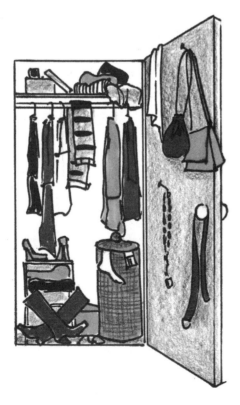

While the idea of cleaning out your closet may sound like pure torture, it is in fact an excellent opportunity to practice the Rules of Camouflage Chic. As you're sorting through and trying on various clothing (a necessary part of the project), give some serious thought as to why a particular outfit makes you look heavier or slimmer than another. What rules are being broken or followed? Is the fabric too shiny or the collar too big? Or is there a slimming vertical line just where you need it? This kind of conscious thought process truly fine-tunes your style sense. By the time your closet's organized and you're ready for your next serious shopping expedition, you'll find yourself seeing things so clearly that you'll be able to zip through the stores like a professional stylist.

Cleaning Out Your Closet

THE PREP

First you'll need a few **basics:**

1. One or two portable hanging racks. Those nice big ones you see being wheeled around department stores would be perfect, but smaller, cheaper ones will do. You can find perfectly adequate racks for between fifteen and forty dollars at places such as Hold Everything, bed and bath stores, or huge home supply warehouses like Home Depot.
2. Some of those lovely white cardboard storage boxes with cutout handles that come packaged six for seven dollars at office supply stores.
3. Tissue paper or plastic dry cleaner bags to ensure wrinkle-free storage.

You also may need some clear plastic stacking boxes and a shoe holder, but wait to do a full assessment before purchasing these.

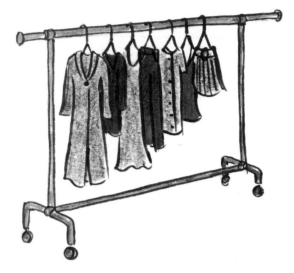

Next, you'll need some **time.** So set aside anywhere from a few hours to a few days to plow through, sort out, and try on your clothes and organize your closet. Base the organization time on the magnitude and state of your wardrobe. How long has it been since you've explored the deeper recesses of your closet? How big a mess is it in there? My mess rarely takes more than a few hours to pull back into shape since I have a low tolerance for clutter. My friend Betsy, on the other hand . . . well, last time I visited we spent a good twenty minutes searching under piles of clothes for the mate to a particular shoe before we finally gave up. I've never seen anything like it! I'd say Betsy has a couple of good solid days' work there—if not a week. But even then it's not necessarily painful work. It's rejuvenating and liberating and actually kind of fun when you approach it with a brave new millennium spirit. Just think how lucky you are to have a unique and glorious opportunity to meet a new century fully together and utterly organized. You get a chance like that only once every hundred years!

THE PROJECT

The best approach is to get **everything out of your closet.** If you have two racks, it would be ideal to transfer everything to one of them, but if you have only one just lay everything on the bed or floor. Then start trying on each and every garment one by one. Pieces that fit perfectly and are 100 percent ready to wear go back into the closet. Items that are totally unsalvageable (e.g., old stretched-out sweaters, silk blouses with perspiration stains, etc.) get tossed in the trash or sent to flood victims in third world countries. Garments that are poor quality, itch, or are in oversupply (T-shirts?) or that you know you'll never wear again go into a tax-deductible charity pile. Things that need alteration go in another pile. High-quality gems that don't fit at the moment but you're *sure* will fit, once you lose that extra four and a half pounds, either get hung in a spare closet or covered storage rack or carefully folded between tissue or plastic dry cleaner bags and packed away in storage boxes. (Make sure the boxes are labeled—something like

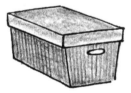

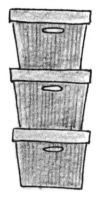

"Skinny Clothes" should do it. Put a date on them, too.) Questionable garments—those you still like but haven't worn much and those you're just not sure about—go on a portable rack for further scrutiny. (This will probably be your biggest section.) That's phase one.

PHASE TWO

Everything should now be off the bed (or first rack). Good clothes are back in the closet, others are in neat little piles on the floor, some are boxed up—labeled and gone—and the rest are on the portable rack. Now realistically scrutinize everything on the rack—what's the story with this stuff? Something's wrong with it or it would already be back in the closet with your favorite clothes. So what's the problem? Is it a style or color you would never dream of wearing again now that you're into camouflage? Was it a mistake in the first place? Is the silhouette fattening? Is it dated and you're just hanging on to it because you wore it the night you were voted prom queen? Or maybe you could just never figure out quite what to do with it—sometimes it's not the garment itself that's bad, but rather what you've been wearing it with.

Try combining different tops with different bottoms. Try various-shape tops under jackets or over other tops. Maybe you need to buy something to complete one of the outfits—if so, start a shopping list. See if any of the pieces on the rack complements any of the choice pieces you've put back in the closet. Experiment with accessories. You might just come up with something great. Finally, hang all acceptable clothing back in your closet with your perfect pieces. Then have a yard sale to get rid of whatever's left on the rack—or give it away to friends, relatives, or charity.

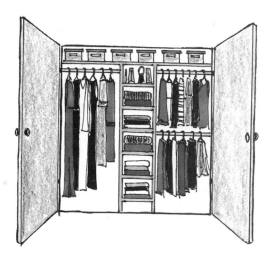

NEXT STEP

Are we having fun yet? Hang your pared-down wardrobe in your closet according to garment type first, color second, then shape. This plan would have all jackets hanging together in one section, trousers in another, dresses, tops, vests, etc. in their own sections. Within those sections items are arranged according to color: neutrals first, dark to light—starting with black, ending in creams and whites—and lastly your brights. And within those color sections, black tops, for instance, are the shapes—all V necks together, or all mock turtles, or whatever. Don't forget—in the summer move your heavy winter-only pieces to another closet or onto a covered hanging storage rack. Do the same with your lightest-weight summer-only things in the winter.

YOUR DRESSER

Now move along to your **dresser.** Throw out all old underwear, stockings with runs, single socks, and bras that don't fit. Be brutal. New underwear is an affordable luxury and always a pick-me-up (literally, as well as figuratively). Think about storing sea-

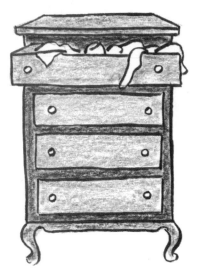

sonal things such as thermal underwear in nice plastic see-through storage bins. Write a list as you go of what needs to be replenished, then go out *within the week* and buy it, so it will be there when you need it. Make sure you have surplus panty hose in the right tones, the right-style bras for all your tops, fresh white socks for the gym. You know the drill.

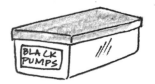

ACCESSORIES

Now go through the same process with your **accessories.** Shoes that are stored in boxes should either be labeled or moved into clear plastic stackable boxes. Those that are unboxed should be arranged according to style and color—all black dressy heels here, all brown sporty shoes there, either on the closet floor or in a hanging shoe organizer. **Get rid of old shoes that don't fit** (feet change size as we age). Store those you simply can't part with but will seldom (if ever) wear in another white storage box, labeled and dated, of course. Jewelry should be out of little cardboard boxes and easy to see—neatly arranged in either a large jewelry box, clear plastic divided boxes, or baskets. Belts should be hanging together or in clear boxes. And there you have it. **You're a new person!** You may even lose a few ounces doing this!

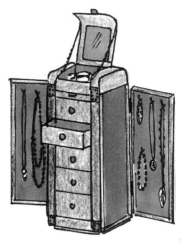

4

SHOPPING, ALTERATIONS, AND BATHING SUITS (EEK!)

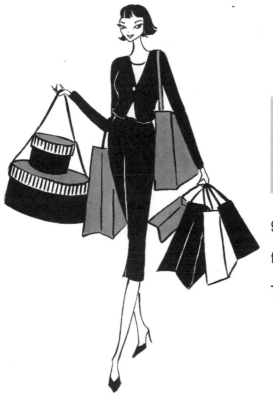

People in stores don't care if you go out looking like a bumblebee, they just want to sell the garment. They don't care how you look.

—ROB KINCH, custom designer

N ow that you know the kinds of things you want in your wardrobe, all you have to do is find them. This is the fun part—or not—depending on your relationship with shopping, which can be as complex as the one you have with your mother. Some women are shopaholics who suffer severe withdrawal symptoms if there are no stores within a three-mile radius. Others are mallophobic and consider shopping more torturous than a trip to the dentist. Most of us, though, fall somewhere in between—we get a major adrenaline rush when we find something that's totally perfect at an incredible price and are considerably less euphoric about the entire process when we end up empty-handed after hours of try-ons and slogging through crowds.

Hitting the jackpot and coming up with a little treasure is partly luck and partly timing—especially if you're a sale shopper—but it's also a good part shopping savvy and solid strategies, too. A little planning will increase your chances of finding what you want tenfold and make shopping more fun and less stressful. Here, then, are the shopping strategies to live by. Think of them as the *inner game of shopping*. It adds a nice spiritual touch to the whole thing.

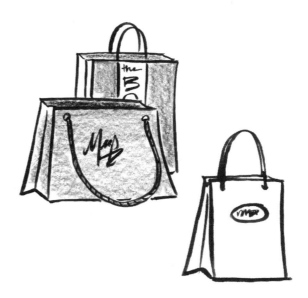

THE INNER GAME OF SHOPPING

• **Shop alone** (or with a professional consultant who is *totally* dedicating her time to shop with you). Don't listen to anyone who tells you it's better to shop with friends. It's not. Successful shopping requires a certain amount of focus—especially now that you'll be concentrating on specific slimming lines, shapes, silhouettes, colors, etc. Friends and relatives present too much of a distraction, and if they haven't read this book,

they won't entirely get what it is you're looking for anyway. You need time on your own to experiment and to learn to trust your own instincts.

In general, other people's opinions are essentially a reflection of their own image and tastes—and what's good for them might not be good for you. Plus, everybody sees you in a different light. Mom might still see you as her little girl. Your loving husband might think you look good in everything or have a hard time visualizing a fully accessorized finished look. And friends will probably see you as you are now—not the new and improved Camouflage Chic version you're aiming for. It's all too risky. Even with the best of intentions, it's almost impossible for shopping partners to be totally objective. Go it alone. Take your time. Enjoy.

• **Shop on high-energy days** when you're feeling fresh and energetic and have plenty of time. Do not shop under the influence of PMS or menopausal blues. You don't want to break down in tears when the saleslady says she's out of your size. Plus, your hormones will tell you you're fat and ugly and nothing looks good on you anyway, except possibly a $3,500 Chanel suit.

- **Plan ahead.** If you need something for a special occasion, don't wait till the last minute, or even the last day, to shop. Unless there's a star in the east, you won't find what you want. You'll wind up settling for something that's just okay, wear it once, and be stuck with another albatross in the closet. Give yourself time. If you do find yourself in a last-minute dilemma, let your fingers do the walking. Call the best store in your area, ask for your favorite salesperson, the personal shopper, or the manager and describe what you're looking for. If they've got some possibilities, ask them to pull them for you, then zip in for a quick try-on. There are no guarantees that you'll find exactly what you want, but you've got a better shot than rushing around all over creation.

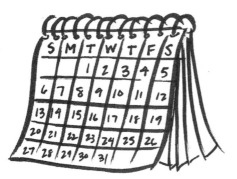

- **Try not to compromise.** Don't buy something unless you really love it and it is 100 percent slimming. And if you really love it and it's perfect, don't be deterred by price. You get so much more wear from something you love and that suits you perfectly that it's worth whatever you pay for it. If you absolutely must buy something that is less than ideal, at least don't overpay—that way you won't feel guilty disposing of it when you find the perfect replacement.

- **Use the three-way mirrors** in dressing rooms. If there is no three-way mirror, whip out your compact for a rear view. Back and side views are just as important as front ones.

- **Buy multiples.** When you find a garment that is the *perfect* size and shape for you, consider buying a few of them in different colors—or even a backup in the same color. I'm talking primarily about basics like T's, blouses, sweaters, pants, shoes, etc., *not* lush designer ensembles. Ideally, you would wear a potential gem a few times to get a feel for it and see if it measures up to your expectations—and then go buy a few more. But if you think you'll be too busy to get back to the store soon, stock up on the spot. If the item turns out to be not quite the marvel you thought it was, return the unworn backups. Which brings us to the next point: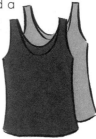

- **Shop in stores with user-friendly return policies.** If you find something you sort of like but it's not perfect—repeat, *perfect*—make sure it's returnable. You don't want any more duds in your closet than you already have. Save receipts, it makes life easier.

- **If you find a good salesperson, stick with her.** Make friends. A good salesperson is indispensable. She can not only lead you in the right direction and get you other sizes while you are in the dressing room—as opposed to your running out half dressed to rummage through the racks again—but she can often negotiate for free alterations. Plus, once she knows your style and what a lovely person you are, she will probably be happy to call you when your kind of thing goes on sale.

Remember, though, that salespeople are just like the rest of the population—**they either get it or they don't.** If a salesperson says, "This is what they're all wearing now, dear" or "We sell a lot of these" or tells you how *mahvelous* you look in *everything* you try on, trust me, she doesn't get it.

Just recently, as a case in point, I was shopping for an outfit for a TV spot I was doing. The producer had wanted me to wear something in gray to complement the set. The saleswoman kept telling me that I looked just fabulous in every little gray number I tried on. Some of them did look okay and definitely suited the purpose, but they did not look half as good on me as another color would have. A *good* saleswoman would have at least suggested another more flattering color. Mine didn't, and she had no idea I was locked into gray. *She didn't get it.*

- **Take advantage of personal shoppers.** Most good department stores have them on staff and their services are *free.* You call ahead, tell them what you're looking for, and they'll scout the store and have things gathered for you to try on when you come in. Like salespeople and psychiatrists, though, **some personal shoppers are bound to be better than others.** So feel them out, see if their taste jibes with yours. But don't reject things out of hand in the beginning. Unless the clothes they bring in are *totally* off base, at least try them on. You never know—a personal shopper might open the door to a winning new style for you. In any case, never feel obliged to buy something just because she has gone to the trouble of helping you. It's her job. If you like her and continue to use her services, you will eventually end up buying—when the merchandise is perfect for you.

- **Dress comfortably but well.** Obviously you don't want to be dressed to the hilt for shopping, but it's a good idea not to be in total shlump mode ei-

ther. Wear at least a little makeup, good foundation garments, and casual clothes that are easy to put on and take off. (Take along a pair of heels if you're shopping for clothes that require them.) In winter, check your coat or leave it in the car. If worse comes to worst and you have to lug it around, toss it in an extra shopping bag. (I actually pack an ultralightweight nylon shoulder strap tote in my purse—it weighs practically nothing and folds into a tiny square.) You need both hands free for ultimate shopping.

- **Take a swatch if you're trying to match.** All you really need is a tiny little piece cut from a seam allowance.

- **Shop by process of elimination.** Now that you know the colors, textures, lines, and shapes that are best for you, don't waste your time checking out every piece of merchandise in the store. Zero in on color first, then check for style and fabric. This is particularly useful in discount stores where the occasional gem is mixed in with beaucoup garbage. Cruise through, stop when you spot one of your colors, look, feel, try on or move on.

- **Take your time.** Don't shop when you're in a rush. Rushing causes mistakes.

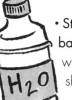

- **Stick a small bottle of water in your bag.** (I'm never without one.) Often when you feel tired or hungry while shopping, it's dehydration.

- **Scout the stores whenever you can.** It's easier to make more frequent forays than go for a whole exhausting day of shopping. It's like grazing instead of gulping a big meal. Also, familiarity breeds *content*—knowing where everything is and getting to know various salespeople make shopping much less daunting.

- **Shop during the week if possible.** The stores are packed on weekends and it's one line after another . . . plus, it's very hard to get salespeople to help you.

- **Examine the fit with a critical eye** (see Rule 5). Think about what can be easily altered and what cannot (I'll talk more about this in the next section). For instance, if you find a great jacket on sale but the lapels are a little too wide, you might want to think about getting them fixed. Too low an armhole, on the other hand, would be too difficult and costly to fix.

- **Even if you're budget conscious, cruise through the haute couture collections** and top-of-the-line casual departments *first* so that you have a good feel for quality and current trends. This is called *comparison shopping.* Don't be intimidated by costs or snooty saleswomen. If they were royalty they would not be working at the store, they'd be yachting on the Riviera.

- **When budget is an issue, shop the sales.** Sales are the perfect time to refurbish and update your basics—those timeless staples that are the core of your wardrobe. Sales are not the time, on the other hand, to buy trendy fad items, since the fad will be dead or rapidly dying by the time you pull out your credit card. Best sales times: before and after holidays; January for clearance of fall and winter outerwear and accessories; July for summer clothes and shoes.

- **Resist going for a great deal just because it's a great deal.** Even if the discount is substantial, it's no bargain if you never wear it. This is a trap that snags the best of us—especially in outlet stores. Watch it!

- **Always ask nicely for an extra discount if a garment is flawed in any way.** You'll most always get it.

Shopping for me is torture—torture! I'm missing a female gene or something.

—GLORIA ESTEFAN, singer

ALTERED STATES: WHAT CAN, AND CANNOT, BE ALTERED

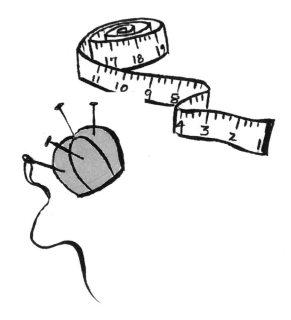

Mass-market clothing—and that includes everything from designer pret-a-porter to Kmart kouture—is sized to fit the largest number of people most of the time in whatever specific demographic the line is targeting. **If you fall outside the norm in any way, you will probably need the occasional nip and tuck to make a garment fit properly.** New York custom designer Rob Kinch, who specializes in chic custom-made clothing that slims and trims, estimates that while 75 percent of women who buy retail *think* the clothes they buy fit them, only 35 percent or less are *actually* getting clothes that fit them the way they should.

Aside from the proportional variances we discussed in Rule 4, Rob points out that a good percentage of our bodies are **asymmetrical.** "It's very common," he says. "When you buy clothing and it doesn't look right on you when you get it home, that's usually why. One side will fit nicely and the other side droops or puckers. Most women either don't realize it or think there's something wrong with them. But it's just human physiology; nobody's perfect on both sides. A lot of the models that walk down the runway aren't perfect on both sides either. It can be hips, shoulders, arm length, even bust sizes . . . one breast is usually a different size than the other, and if you're doing a fitted garment, you have to work around it."

While Rob would be happy to make you impeccable custom clothes that fit every little asymmetric part of you to a T (and you can reach him at 212-629-4633), most of us will still be buying the majority of our clothing off the rack—and probably, at least some of the time, at stores that don't offer alterations. That means that sooner or later we'll need the services of a tailor or seamstress. The real trick is finding a good one. Truly talented tailors are rare. Almost any tailor can handle simple up-and-down and in-and-out adjustments, **but only the best of them come up with creative solutions and are able to deal with matters of balance and drape.**

A good tailor, for instance, wouldn't think of just sewing along the outside seams when narrowing the legs on a pair of trousers. He (or she) would understand that the crease would then be thrown off center and ruin the drape. Your average tailor wouldn't much care.

Unfortunately, other than perhaps word of mouth, there is really no 100 percent foolproof way to tell how good a tailor is until you start working with him, but there are a few telltale signs to look for. For one, a good tailor *listens* to you and can explain what he plans to do to solve the problem. If he doesn't want to take the time to do that, or interrupts and talks over you, or is dismissive, try another tailor.

You can also learn a lot by watching a tailor with other customers. I once noticed that one particular tailor I used to go to had no opinion whatsoever when a customer, whose skirt she was pinning, asked her what length she felt was right. To me it was quite obvious what length was best. Why didn't the tailor know? I wished I had consciously registered her lackluster response and just walked out. Instead, I left her a brand-new silk vest to alter, which she subsequently ruined. Live and learn.

For any kind of alteration other than a simple hemming, you've probably got a better shot at excellence at a tailor or dressmaker shop, as opposed to your local dry cleaner. Not to say there are no good tailors at those little worktables in the windows. I'm sure there must be, but dry cleaners are about dry cleaning and tailoring shops are about tailoring, so if you're starting out your search cold it just makes more sense to start with the specialists. Once you've found somebody who seems reliable, proceed with caution! Bring in only one or two things to start with and see what kind of work he does. Don't put your entire wardrobe at risk at one time—it could prove disastrous.

As for what can and can't be altered, here's the scoop according to my experts: Rob, whom you know, and Manuel, Nashville's custom designer to the country music stars and tailor extraordinaire. Some alterations, they say, are easy, some are possible but labor-intensive, and some are impossible.

Easy to Do

- Shortening pants, skirts, jackets, dresses, and sleeves. One notable exception here: hemming bias-cut garments is extremely tricky. It takes experience and a very delicate hand. You need a real pro for this operation. Also, when hemming jackets, keep a close watch on where the pockets fall and the overall proportion. It's usually risky to hem a jacket more than an inch or so.

- Taking in waists on pants or skirts and seats on pants.

- Letting out waists, if not more than an inch or so.

- Nipping in the waist of a jacket to give you a little more shape.

- Tapering a sleeve (if the armhole is right).

- Removing pant pockets.

- Tapering a straight skirt. (If you still want to be able to walk, two inches is about max for a taper.)

Tricky to Do

- Reshaping lapels. More labor-intensive than difficult. To do it right, the tailor needs to take the jacket apart. He could cheat, though, by cutting it while it's on the jacket

and stitching it closed with a blind stitch, which would be cheaper. Either way, the tailor needs to be A class.

- Raising an armhole. Manuel says once the armhole is cut, there is no way to make it smaller, except by sewing in a triangular bridge piece, and that works only with dark fabrics where it will be relatively unnoticeable (another plus for dark neutrals).

- Lengthening a sleeve when there is not enough extra fabric in the hem. One way around this is to add a new piece of fabric. The trick, however, is to proportion it properly and perhaps even add piping or some kind of trim (in the same color) where it is attached to make it look like part of the design.

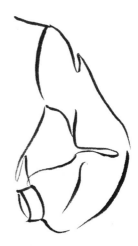

Impossible to Do

- Changing the pant rise. *It has to fit.* If it doesn't, there's nothing you can do about it except give the pants away.

- Letting out silk, rayon, or velvet garments. The original stitching line always shows on fragile fabrics like these, says Manuel. Don't do it.

Costs

Alteration costs will vary from tailor to tailor and neighborhood to neighborhood. Other considerations such as fabric and design of the garment are also factored in. In general, **the trickier the alteration, the costlier the procedure.** The following prices represent a good average basis (this year, anyway): pants hemmed—$10 to $20; sleeves hemmed—$8 to $25; skirts hemmed—$15 to $40; shoulders narrowed or reset—$40 to $120; waist nipped—$30; pants or skirt tapered—$10 to $40; jacket narrowed—$35 to $110 (the more vertical seams in the jacket, the easier it will be to alter).

Whether or not a garment is worth altering depends on the quality of the piece and your attachment to it. It might be worth narrowing the jacket of a vintage eighties Valentino power suit, but probably not an old worn-out Gap jacket. Obviously, *perfect* fit is much less of an issue in knock-around clothing than it is with your serious prime pieces.

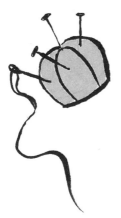

Custom Clothes

Yes! If you can afford it, custom design is a fabulous way to go, at least for a few timeless basics. The *less* evenly proportioned your body, the harder you are to fit, the more you should consider this route. Your clothes will fit perfectly! Custom designer prices vary. Rob's jackets and dresses go for approximately $1,000 and trousers, skirts, and blouses between $450 and $550, depending on the fabric. Other designers are probably in the same ballpark. When you think about it, though, it's actually *less* than a lot of designers' off-the-rack prices—*and it will fit as if it was made for you . . .* because it was.

There are also tailors and seamstresses (not *designers*, like Rob) who will copy your favorite garment in the fabric of your choice. They will even make slight alterations along the way, so that the new garment may fit *better* than the original. This is one of my sister Eda's favorite routes. "I had a fabulous blazer that I loved," she says, "but it was worn and I had gained weight. So I took it to a tailor, along with some fabric I had bought, and she copied it, giving me a couple of extra inches. The end product was so successful, I ended up getting several made in different fabrics for day and evening." Prices for custom copies again will vary, but a jacket will probably cost between $300 and $400 if you bring in your own fabric.

BATHING SUITS: SHOPPING AND CAMOUFLAGING TIPS

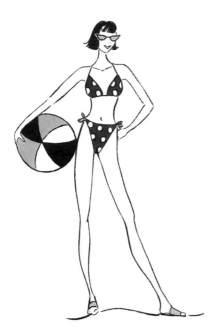

Swimsuits are, of course, in a class by themselves: one of the **least fun things to shop for—and impossible to alter.** Bathing-suit shopping puts you between grim reality and horrid overhead fluorescence—frankly, not one of my favorite places to be. Still, if you want to frolic in the sea and surf you're going to need a suit—and it might as well be one that flatters.

> I'm not in my element standing around in a bikini in front of strangers. I never stand up in a bikini, even at the swimming pool. I feel like a normal person when it comes to things like that. I'm like any other girl who doesn't want to show her bottom.
>
> —ELIZABETH HURLEY, actress/model/producer

Actually, Elizabeth Hurley has discovered one of the best bathing-suit camouflage strategies yet—*don't stand up!* Another tactic along the same lines would be to do all your sunning on the Black Sea at some Crimean resort, where you would look positively undernourished in comparison to the locals. Probably more practical, though, is a sarong (see Rule 6 for wrap ideas) or a roomy ultra-lightweight gauzy cotton shirt—actually, both are always good to have on standby as emergency sun protectors anyway. But choreography, geography, and full cover-ups aside, there are a few ways to improve your chances of looking good in a swimsuit:

- **Give yourself time to shop.** This is extremely important with swimwear. You have to try on *a lot* of suits. You'd be surprised how suits that look so similar can fit so differently. **Try styles you might not ordinarily consider**—sometimes they work better than you think. And of course, as always, look for designs that will accentuate your positives and visually eliminate the negatives. If you have a lovely bosom and heavy hips, make sure the bodice of the suit is perfectly well cut and gorgeous and the bottom unobtrusive

- Look for Suitable Solutions hang tags, which many manufacturers now have on their suits. They can be of some help in pinpointing a suit's benefits. The tag lists six features (bust minimizer, bust maximizer, full-cup support, tummy/midriff toner, long torso, hip/thigh maximizer) with a little hole next to each; when the hole is punched out, the suit has that particular feature. It's not an exact science, but it's a good start.

- **Always try at least one size larger** than you think you wear. When suits are tight, the edges cut into any excess flesh and make bulges. Suits that fit a bit looser compress flesh less—hence nothing is squeezed, nothing pops out.

- **Look for high Lycra content.** The more Lycra in the suit, the more it will hold you in.

- **Check the inside construction.** Some suits have hidden features such as underwire bra support, bust enhancers, double linings, or tummy-trimming panels that could serve you well.

- **Stick to the darker colors or tones close to your skin color**—remember that dark colors recede, making the figure appear smaller, and skin-tone suits give the impression of an all-over monotone, always a winner.

- **No big prints.** Small or sparse prints are okay, but big prints pop out, making you look bigger. If you can't resist, at least make sure you wear the print where it will draw attention *away* from problem areas. A print top paired with a matching solid bottom, for instance, would draw attention away from hips and thighs.

- **Cleverly placed vertical and diagonal stripes and/or color blocks can help slim.** Placement

on the suit and where the stripes or blocks fall on your body are key. The only way to know for sure if they're in the right place for *your* body is to try it on.

- **No shiny fabrics**—every bump shows in reflective fabrics! You need a little *texture* to help conceal little bulges.

- **Shirring across the front of a suit can camouflage tummies,** but watch that the style isn't too dowdy.

- **Go for the highest-cut leg that you feel comfortable in.** The high cut gives the leg more length. Skirted suits and styles with old-fashioned front panels like Esther Williams used to wear make legs look shorter and you stockier. Forget about them. ***And no boy legs!*** Every iota of excess flesh is squeezed down and pops out right where the suit leg ends. They are deadly! If you like the idea of bottoms that resemble shorts, make sure they are *wide* around the thigh.

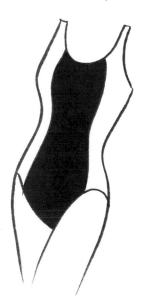

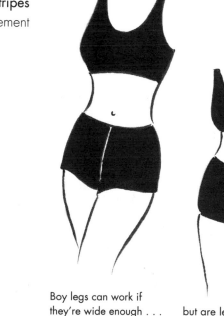

Boy legs can work if they're wide enough . . .   but are lethal if they're too tight

- For ex–bikini wearers who have developed tummies—you can still wear a two-piece, just try a higher-waisted brief with a nice high-cut leg and plenty of spandex.

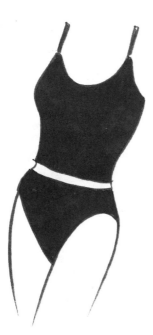

- **Watch the size of pads in underwire push-up bras.** Unless you're ultra-small-busted, either take them out or replace them with smaller ones. Most of the time they look unnatural—and they stay wet longer than the rest of the suit.

- **Short-waisted women** sometimes have a hard time finding one-piece suits that are short enough in the torso. **For a one-piece look try a "tank-ini"**—a tank top and high-waisted bikini bottom. (This is my personal favorite.)

- If you're a totally different size on top and bottom, look for a label that sells tops and bottoms **separately.** Make sure, though, that you buy tops and bottoms that are in proportion. A little skimpy bikini top paired with a big full bottom, for instance, would look out of balance.

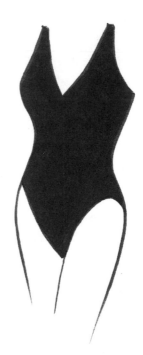

- **Full-busted women** obviously need suits with good support. Look for underwire bra support and/or high Lycra content. Also try suits sized for long torsos, since your bust dimension can use up the extra fabric meant for a longer waist.

- **Re thong bikinis:** Listen to *Sports Illustrated*'s bathing-suit model Kathy Ireland: "They're not very comfortable, they look good on very few people, plus your butt gets all sunburned."

> *At Sports Illustrated we would try on hundreds [of suits]. It's important to find one that complements your body and not try to fit into something that doesn't work.*
>
> —KATHY IRELAND, **model**

5

LAST, SOME CAMOUFLAGING TIPS FOR HIM

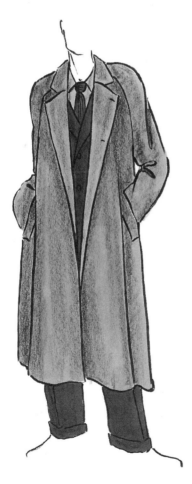

A good man often appears *gauche* simply because he does not take advantage of the myriad mean little chances of making himself look stylish. Preferring truth to form, he is not constantly at work upon the façade of his appearance.

—IRIS MURDOCH, British novelist, philosopher

S ince "Does this make me look fat?" is really a cross-gender question, I really couldn't leave you without a little something to share with the man—or men—in your life. Men care about all this too, they're just usually a little more reluctant to ask about it—probably for the same reason they never ask for directions . . . but then that's another book. Also, since you're most likely the one who serves as general counsel on all things sartorial anyway, you should have this info under your belt (or at least at your fingertips—we don't want to ruin your line). Then the next time he asks, "Does this make me look fat?" you can provide the definitive answer.

> I don't mind that I'm fat. You still get the same money.
>
> —MARLON BRANDO, actor

In general, most of the Rules of Camouflage Chic apply to men, too. Okay, maybe not the parts about foundation garments, panty hose, and stiletto heels, but a substantial part of the rest of the information. Dark colors, similar tones, and monochromes, for instance, are just as slimming for men. So are vertical and diagonal lines, nonbulky fabrics, good proportional balance, and the principles of understated elegance. So a lot of what you already know can be applied to your guys as well.

But there are some specifics that are particularly male-oriented. So let's get to them, starting with suits.

SUITS

Design choice is always a matter of personal style. But for the majority of men—leaving aside avant-garde types and European dandies—the most flattering suit shape is one that is neither too relaxed and shapeless (à la your standard old Brooks Brothers sack suit prototype), nor too form-fitting and constricting (like ultra-European designs). Look for styles that combine the best of both worlds—the snappier fit of the European cut with the softness and comfort of the All-American style. That means a suit with **a gently tapered waistline, good shoulder definition, and moderately high, but comfortable, armholes.**

As for detailing:

• Watch that **lapels** aren't too skimpy or too wide. A good medium width is approximately 3½ inches, which should extend just a fraction less than the halfway mark between the shirt collar and shoulder line. *Wider lapels will make a man look wider.*

• In general, **flap pockets** are more appropriate on a dressy suit—even though they will add a hint of extra dimension to the hip. Patch pockets are fine for sports jackets and sporty suits. *Slit pockets make for the slimmest look.*

- Be aware of back **vents.** They make a big difference in the way a jacket looks, sits, and moves. Of the three basic choices—nonvented, single-vented, or double-vented—most menswear specialists agree that the **double side vents, typically found in English suits, make the body look the slimmest** (unless a man is particularly broad in the beam, in which case he would probably be best off with a single vent). The reason side vents make a man look taller is because the vents visually extend the leg line past the jacket hem, allowing for more movement and fluidity. They also keep the buttocks covered when the hands are in the pockets and don't crease as easily when a man sits. Watch that vents aren't cut too high. The top of the vents, according to tailors, should correspond to the bottom of the pocket flap (which is approximately seven to nine inches up from the hem on a size forty regular jacket).

> *My arms are too short and my torso is too long. I compensate by picking clothes that make my shoulders seem broader and my waist thinner to create a classic V shape.*
>
> —JOHNATHON SCHAECH, actor

Fit

Bad fit can make a man look fat and out of proportion just as easily as it can a woman. (Equality at last!) Although store tailoring is traditionally free for men, store tailors are not out to remake a suit. **Basically, the fewer the alterations they have to make, the happier they are.** In other words, you can't really count on them to point out fit problems. You have to know the basics.

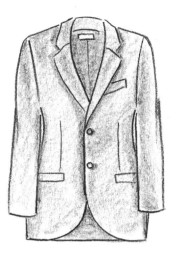

JACKETS

The most crucial areas in a jacket are the *shoulder, chest, armholes,* and *length.* If the first three areas don't fit well when a man first tries on a jacket, they never will. They are, for the most part, **unalterable.** Jacket length can be altered within an inch or two. But more than that throws the jacket, suit, and body out of proportion. So jacket length has to be fairly close to start. Here's how a good jacket should fit:

- **Shoulders** should be wide enough. If they're not, you get an unsightly pull and bulge across the biceps. You want the sleeve to fall perfectly straight from the shoulder with no bumps or pulls.

- The jacket should be **broad enough across the chest** to feel totally comfortable when buttoned. Test by sitting down with the jacket buttoned.

- **Armholes should be cut high enough** that the lower parts fits comfortably up into the armpit but *can't* be felt. Bigger armholes (and sleeves) make a man look dumpy, and the sleeves will bind when the arms are raised.

- **The correct length of a suit jacket is just long enough to cover the bottom of the buttocks. The** usual way of judging length—by dropping arms and aligning the hem with the halfway point of the hand—is not always accurate because arm lengths vary from man to man. (Jackets should be a little longer on tall men for balance.)

While trying on jackets, men should wear a dress shirt to gauge proper sleeve length and collar height. Traditionally, about one-half inch of the shirt collar should show above the jacket, and about one-half inch of shirt cuff should peek out from the sleeve.

The following points make a big difference in how a suit or sports jacket looks—and they are very easy areas to alter.

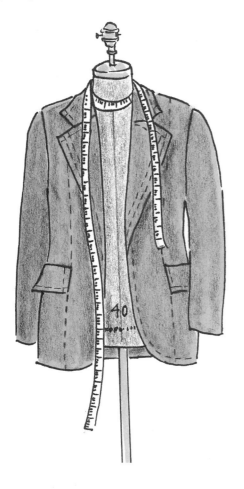

- The jacket **collar** should curve smoothly around the back of the neck, while the lapels lie *flat* on the chest.
- The jacket **waist** should be *slightly* tapered. Jackets with no tapering tend to look a bit boxy. Too much tapering makes the vents pull.
- **Sleeves** should fall to the point where the wrist and hand meet when the arms are hanging naturally by the sides. When getting sleeves altered, make sure the tailor measures both arms, since arm lengths can differ. (I once worked with a male model, a former minor league pitcher, whose right arm was a full three inches longer than his left one!)

TROUSERS

- Always wear shoes when getting pants hemmed. Cuffed trousers should be hemmed in a straight line and be long enough to break slightly over the shoe (about one-half inch over the instep).

- Standard cuff measurement is 1⅝ inches for average men and 1¾ inches for tall men. Pants with no cuffs should be hemmed at a slant so that the back falls slightly lower—to where the heel and sole meet.

- Trousers should be worn *on the waist,* not on the hips like jeans or falling off the hips à la hip-hoppers and your occasional plumber. They not only hang much better when worn in their proper position, they make potbellies much less noticeable.

- Trousers should taper gradually from hip to ankle. Forget about flares, bell-bottoms, and totally straight leg pants—they make short men look shorter.

- The crotch should be as high up as is comfortable. Sagging crotches make a man look dumpy and shorter.

- There should be no pulling across the front pockets or at the pleats. There needs to be enough fullness in the thigh that pleats hang straight and don't open. Pockets should lay flat.

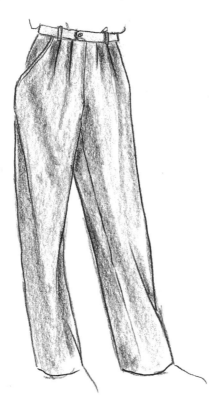

I like a [high-cut] Hollywood waist, though I know that's not really in right now. Everybody likes a more narrow cut, but you have to be a skinny little kid to wear that stuff.

—MATT DILLON, actor

SHIRTS, COLLARS, AND FACE SHAPES

Since shirt collars are an extension of a man's face, they can not only visually reshape his face but also have a huge impact on his entire look. So you want to get it right. Basic collar shape choices are

1. the long straight-point collar
2. the spread collar
3. the button-down
4. the tab collar
5. the Eton collar (which requires a collar pin)
6. the band collar

For the most part, you want to choose collar style according to *face shape* and *neck length*. A good basic rule of thumb when matching face shape to collar is "Opposites attract": Round-faced men do better with angular collars, long narrow faces are better with wider collars. Neck lengths work the other way around: short necks need short collars, long necks need higher collars. With that in mind:

- Short neck—low band collars, collars that lie flat.
- Long thin necks—higher band collars or tab collars.
- Thin elongated faces—medium to wide spread collar.
- Round face—medium to long straight-point or narrow spread collar.
- Short or squat neck or big round face—no small or spread collar, no button-downs. Try pointy collars. Any rounded collar will only accentuate a round face.
- Medium-sized faces and necks—medium-sized collars.

General Tips

- **Double-breasted suits** are dressier and always look better buttoned—on either the top button or the bottom one, not both. Shorter men get a longer line by buttoning only the bottom button. In general, though, a single-breasted suit is more slimming on most men.

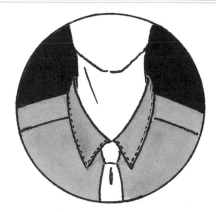

long straight-point collar

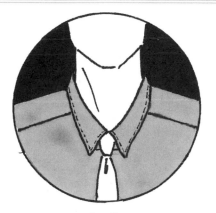

tab collar

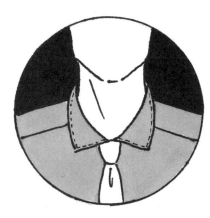

spread collar

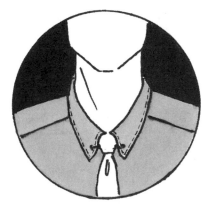

Eton collar

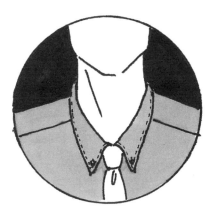

button-down collar

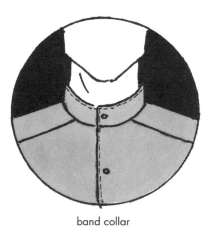

band collar

- **Sports jackets** follow the same fit rules as suit jackets but can be fit a **little looser** to accommodate sweaters.

- **Topcoat length:** Just below the knee is the shortest any man should ever go. If a coat is too short, the proportion shifts and the body looks boxy, stunted, and bulky. The chicest length is probably six to eight inches below the knee, but of course that has to suit a man's individual proportions.

- Big shiny **belt buckles** bring attention to the stomach—men are better off with subtle nonornamental buckles on narrow belts not more than 1¼ inches wide. The right length counts, too—belts shouldn't extend more than a few inches past the first loop nor be so short they hardly make it through the buckle. As for cowboys and their beloved rodeo buckles . . . well, look, they're not slimming, but they are rather quaint in that old out-West kind of way.

- **Ties have to be the right length.** After being tied, the tips of the tie should reach the waistband of the trousers (another reason not to wear trousers on the hips!).

- **Go for nonbulky fabrics.** Corduroys and tweeds add girth. Suits should be made of fine-weave natural fibers, blends, or first-class man-mades. Fabrics should feel soft and have a fabulous drape to them.

- Bigger heads require wider shoulders.

- Men with substantial middles should pass on sweaters with full bands across the stomach.

- Very-wide-legged trousers work only on tall men. Short men are better off with a standard to narrow leg.

- Three- and even four-button suits can make a man look longer and lankier—but they have to suit his

character. They can be a bit trendy. So make sure they are in sync with the man's personality.

- No big shoes with narrow-bottom pants—especially wide squarish ones.

- Avoid big dopey overlarge jackets. Jackets that contour the body are much more slimming and chic.

- No big bold ties with print shirts. Wear them with solids, please. No striped ties with striped shirts.

- Forget about hankies in the pockets; they interrupt the line.

- For formal occasions, men with prominent stomachs should try vests instead of cummerbunds. Anyone who does wear cummerbunds, remember that the pleats are worn up—to catch the crumbs, I'm told.

- Collars on dress shirts should fit snugly without choking or chafing the neck. Too big looks just as bad as too small. The body of the shirt should fit comfortably, without excess material that could gather into little bulges and wreck the line of the jacket. (All-cotton shirts tend to shrink. Add a half inch in sleeve length and collar size when buying.)

EXTRA TIPS FOR HEAVYSET MEN

- Vertical lines like pinstripes are fine. Plaids are definitely out of the question, except *perhaps* for very subtle ones—but why bother? Dark solids are safest.

- Suiting fabric should be smooth, not bulky. Look for the smooth midweight variety with good drape.

- Clothes should be cut generously. Skimpy makes bulges show.

- Jackets should be slightly longer than normal and hang straight down in back. Sleeves should be tapered.

- Trouser bottoms should be just a bit narrower than usual.

- Double-breasted jackets are not advisable, but if they are worn, they are the most slimming when buttoned on the *bottom* button.

- Flat-front pants may be more appropriate. Trousers with pleats should be made so that the pockets are easily accessible, and the trousers should be worn *on the waistline*.

- Men with big bellies might consider **suspenders,** since they allow the pants to hang better (and they don't really show anyway when worn with a jacket). Pants should be a half inch fuller in the waist and a little bit longer when worn with suspenders.

- Shoes should be simple, without a lot of toe decoration.

EXTRA TIPS FOR SHORT MEN

- Buy short sizes. Don't buy regular and shorten—everything will be out of proportion.

- Jacket shoulders should be nice and square, not slouchy.

- Jacket length is crucial—not too long or too short.

- Trousers should be tapered at the bottom a bit more than normal.

- Shoes should not be too delicate.

- Topcoats should not be too long—just below knee length is a good starting point.

CONCLUSION—A FINAL THOUGHT

> *Beauty comes from an intelligent mind. Women should be growing their minds and then they will be beautiful, because they will have more depth and dimension. They'll enjoy life more.*
>
> —EVE LOM, skin-care entrepreneur

We now reach the final frontier of Camouflage Chic: the special qualities that you, and only you, can bring to the fashion equation. Clothes can slim you down, but they are far from the entire picture. It's your unique spirit—your tastes, attitudes, manners, humor, grooming, energy, and carriage—that completes the picture and shapes your personal style. (Be sure to check the Appendix for important posture and fitness info.) *Personal style is the perfect blending of your special qualities with the clothes you choose.* It's the intersection of who you are with what you wear.

> *Fashions fade, style is eternal.*
>
> —YVES SAINT LAURENT, designer

So as Camouflage Chic helps you shape and highlight your physical assets, take time to **recog-** nize, acknowledge, and cultivate your less tangible assets. Is your intelligence luminous? The timbre of your voice intriguing? Your smile iridescent? Your humor wonderfully quirky? Your kindness inspiring? Your posture regal? **Don't overlook the sterling qualities that make you unique. Own them. Let them shine.**

If you have a few little rough spots (after all, nobody's perfect), take note and polish them up. Lord knows, if Courtney Love can do it, anyone can. Taking a personal inventory from time to time can actually be rather enlightening when done with objectivity and love. Consider everything from personal grooming habits to attitudes. True women of style are always described by adjectives such as *energetic, determined, good-humored, graceful, charming, witty, humble, vital, colorful, adventurous, dedicated, cultured, effervescent, kind, resourceful, original, fearless, appreciative, optimistic.* I personally find those words inspiring.

"You don't even have to be fashionable to have style," Diana Vreeland once said. "It's just a marvelous thing that people have, and it's something all of their own. It has very little to do with clothes. The clothes just work very well for them." There's no doubt she's right when you think of some of the legendary men and women whose names are synonymous with style: Audrey Hepburn, Jackie O., Katharine Hepburn, Marlene Dietrich, Fred Astaire, Cary Grant, Lauren Bacall, and Ms. Vreeland herself. It's not their clothes we remember so much about them as their personalities, grace, manner of speaking, and attitudes. And the same is true of you.

Great personal style, of course, isn't built in a day. It develops and matures naturally as you become more aware and astute about yourself, others, and fashion in general. Wherever you are on your personal course, the information in this book gives you a foot up. You now know everything you need to know to look slim *and* stylish—when you want to, of course. Chances are you won't play by all the Rules of Camouflage Chic all the time, and to tell you the truth I don't really expect you to. If you're like me, there are times when, to paraphrase Rhett, you frankly just don't give a damn. Who really cares if they look a little chunky mowing the lawn, grocery shopping, or sightseeing on the Ganges? Sometimes it's just plain irrelevant. But when you do care, when looking your absolute best does matter, you can always depend on the Rules of Camouflage Chic. Sure, exceptions to the Rules can work *occasionally.* But the Rules of Camouflage Chic *always* work. They are as solid as a Tiffany diamond.

> *Lots of people have told me I am beautiful. But the one who touched me the most was Stevie Wonder. He can't even see, but he said there was some inner beauty in me that he felt.*
>
> —ERYKAH BADU, singer

APPENDIX—

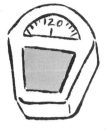

THE LAST WORD ON LOOKING THINNER

Although I wrote this book with an eye toward style and fashion, I would be remiss if I didn't at least mention a few other surefire ways to look slimmer. I think of these as the physical part of Camouflage Chic.

POSTURE

This is your ace in the hole. *Good posture makes everybody look 150 percent better.* It makes you look taller. It makes you look thinner. It makes your clothes hang better. It's probably the most consistent connective thread running through all women of style. There's a certain magnetism, self-confidence, and to-the-manner-born charisma about a strong, graceful carriage. It's body language that works.

> *When I'm conscious of how I'm standing and carrying myself well, everybody says, "Oh, you've lost weight"!*
>
> —DEBORAH KAHAN, choreographer/dancer

But there's much more to good posture than your mother might have told you. You may *think* you're standing up straight, while in fact you are hyperextending your lower lumbar spine, which makes your derriere stick out, or leading with your chin, which can lead to neck and back problems.

The real trick to good posture, according to the experts, is *proper body alignment*—which is *not,* they point out, about tucking in the pelvis, pulling your shoulders back, holding up your head, and stiffening up like a soldier. It's more about aligning your head, ribs, and hips and lifting up from your abdominals, separating your ribs from your hips, and feeling a strong center. In fact, stand up right now and try this little experiment: Stand relaxed with your hands at your side. Visualize your ears centered over your shoulders, your shoulders over your hips, hips over knees (which may necessitate tucking your pelvis a bit), and knees over ankles. Now lift your ribs. It's a very subtle movement, but it makes you taller. I swear it gives me another inch.

BODYWORK METHODS

Home experiments aside, there are a few excellent **bodywork methods** that are wonderful for improving alignment and helping you move with more fluidity. Some of them have been popular with dancers and athletes for years. Now many are becoming downright mainstream—and a lot more available to us civilians.

Yoga

Of all of the bodywork methods, **yoga** is probably the most widely known. It is an excellent exercise for general conditioning and improving posture, although to call yoga an *exercise* doesn't really do it justice. It's more like one-stop shopping for well-being. Yoga combines movement (different poses) with meditation, breathing, and relaxation to integrate and balance mind, body, and soul. Practiced *regularly*, it tones, stretches, and strengthens the body, while at the same time clearing, centering, and calming the mind. **In other words, it nourishes all that makes up the whole person,** which is, no doubt, one of the reasons it has become increasingly popular in the West.

> *Flexibility, besides being an unrivalled aid to good posture, also lengthens the muscles, giving your limbs a longer, leaner look.*
>
> —RAQUEL WELCH, actress, from her book *Raquel: The Raquel Welch Total Beauty and Fitness Program*

Maybe the best thing about yoga is that you can start at any age and do it for your entire lifetime. You can't be too old or too out of shape—your body and your posture will improve no matter what your condition when you start.

Individual or small classes are the best idea if you're just getting started, since your teacher can make corrections in your poses—a simple shift of weight can make a big difference. As in all fields, however, some teachers are better than others. So ask around for a good yoga teacher—this is one place word of mouth really counts. Once you've zeroed in on a worthy prospect, make sure you talk to her or someone at the yoga school to find out the kind of yoga they teach there and if it is appropriate for your level of expertise. If you go to a class and don't enjoy it, try a few others until you find a teacher with whom you connect. Don't give up!

The Internet is a great source for yoga information, and there are many yoga books and tapes available.

> *I recommend that my clients do yoga. It makes you fall in love with yourself.*
>
> —ART LUNA, hair-color superstar

Modern Dance

Modern dance classes are another overall conditioning option that emphasizes posture. They offer a little less spirituality and a lot more peppy music. You'll still get stretched and aerobicized along with body-mind centering. Some classes even have live accompanists, which I've been told can add a whole other dimension to the experience. Definitely worth considering if you can find good classes in your area.

The Pilates Method

Pilates (officially, the Pilates Method of Body Conditioning) improves your posture as it strengthens your body—with emphasis on stomach, back, and derriere. It's really an exercise/alignment hybrid that was developed in the twenties by physical trainer Joseph Pilates. The system is built around a series of controlled exercises that are done on five major pieces of equipment—the Reformer, Cadillac, Barrel, Tower, Chair—and a floor mat. (Some group classes are taught on the mat alone.) Emphasizing body alignment and correct breathing, Pilates uses the abdomen, lower back, and buttocks together as a power center (called "the powerhouse") that enables the rest of the body to move freely. The main goals are muscular harmony, balance, flexibility, and strength for the entire body.

Pilates is taught on a one-to-one basis, or in small groups, by highly trained teachers (to get certified, teachers have to go through seminar training and six hundred apprenticeship hours), so each lesson can be specially geared to your particular capabilities and needs. That makes it ideal for everyone from your grandma to Danny "Lethal Weapon" Glover (who I just heard is a devotee). Joseph Pilates used to tell his students they would "feel better in ten sessions, look better in twenty sessions, and have a completely new body in thirty sessions." I personally felt stronger after one lesson and fully intend to keep it up.

Prices vary according to individual instructors, but they range from thirty-five to sixty dollars each for private lessons and average about ten dollars per group lesson. For more information on Pilates classes or certified trainers in your area, call 800-474-5283 or 800-PILATES.

> Posture is the quickest weight-loss program in the world.
>
> —MARCIA GAY HARDEN, actress

The Alexander Technique

The Alexander Technique is totally about alignment and body awareness; it is not a workout. It was developed in the early 1900s by F. M. Alexander, an Australian actor who had discovered that his constant voice problems were, in fact, caused by his habit of pulling his head back and tightening his neck as he performed. **Today, the technique is based on correcting postural habits.** The heart of the technique lies in the head-neck-body relationship and the elimination of habits that cause tension. Major goals: redefining overall body awareness, lengthening the back, and getting the head and spine balanced and working in harmony. Beneficial side effect: better carriage of the body's weight. The technique is taught one on one, with the teacher making gentle corrections and adjustments.

For a list of certified teachers, call the American Center for the Alexander Technique at 212-799-0468. Private instruction costs between $30 and $125 per hour, depending on location and instructor's credentials.

Feldenkrais Method

The goal of **Feldenkrais,** developed by Moishe Feldenkrais in the 1940s, is much the same as Alexander—body awareness and fluidity of movement. Feldenkrais, a scientist and athlete, drew from Alexander as well as martial arts and biomechanics. Like the Alexander Technique, this is not a workout but a series of lessons geared to differentiate functions of movement. To locate a certified Feldenkrais practitioner near you, call the Feldenkrais Guild at 800-775-2118.

All of these bodywork methods are great for relieving stress and tension—some caused by years, if not decades, of moving, sitting, and standing the wrong way. My theory: If we'd all just had one year of just one of these kinds of body awareness/movement classes in elementary or junior high school, we'd all not only carry ourselves better now but would have far fewer back and neck problems.

You can find more information about any of these methods on the Web. Just type the name—Pilates, Alexander, or Feldenkrais—and let your search engine do the walking. That's how I tracked down my local Pilates teacher. Your local library, alternative newspapers, dance centers, or spas are other good sources for references.

REGULAR EXERCISE

Combine good posture with regular exercise, and you're really cooking. Exercise, of course, helps you look thinner because it helps you *be* thinner. But weight control is only one of its many benefits. It also improves your overall appearance and makes you *feel* better. Regular exercise puts a spring in your walk, increases your energy, decreases stress levels, gives your skin a magic glow, boosts your moods and self-esteem, improves your posture, keeps you young and vital, and, of course, gives you a nice strong body to hang all your new clothes on. It is the panacea of all panaceas.

The pros say that any exercise that counteracts inactivity and boosts your metabolism is good one—even walking up and down stairs instead of taking escalators counts. But all agree that pursuits that include cardiovascular activities, strength training, and flexibility work—and that you can do with some regularity—are ideal. As it turns out, **regularity is the key to it all.** That doesn't mean you have to do the same old exercise all the time—in fact, trainers recommend varying your activities to offset potential injuries as well as boredom. Regularity means actually exercising every day or at least every other day—*not just thinking about doing it.* Because we humans are designed to move a lot, when we don't, we turn to mush. And because our physical energies are so strongly tied to our mental and spiritual well-being, when our physical energy lags, so goes the rest of us . . . and lethargic is not a good look—even in a Chanel.

EATING HABITS/HEALTH

Throughout this book I've mentioned weight only in the most general sense. And that's because I don't really care what you weigh. Some of us are naturally bigger than others. Some have better hair.

Others are better cooks. Diversity keeps things interesting. What I care about is health, not size. If you're big, healthy, and active, terrific. But if your weight is seriously over the top and is making you sluggish and prone to inactivity, you owe it to yourself to get it under control. According to which statistics you go by, somewhere between 22.5 percent and 33.3 percent of Americans are considered obese and are consequently at increased risk for all sorts of chronic diseases, including hypertension, diabetes, arthritis, and a long list of cancers including breast, uterine, cervical, and ovarian. It's not a pretty picture.

So aside from exercising, it's important to eat well, too. Experts worldwide seem to concur that consuming less food is healthier than stuffing ourselves and that a diet high in fruit, veggies, grains, and lean protein is better for us than one full of sugar and fat. There's also considerable evidence that drinking plenty of water keeps the skin clear and the organs healthy and rids the body of toxins, as well as staves off hunger. So take heed. Eat well, drink lots of water, exercise regularly, and stay healthy. Treat your body like the good friend it is. You're worth it. In the long run, health is truly everything. You could have all the money in the world, a closet full of custom couture, and look like Cindy Crawford, and it wouldn't mean a thing without your health.

A sound mind in a sound body, is a short, but full description of a happy state in this world: he that has these two, has little more to wish for; and he that wants either of them, will be little the better for anything else.

—JOHN LOCKE, English philosopher

LET'S KEEP IN TOUCH!

Visit me at

www.LeahFeldon.com

Or call my

consultation hotline

For personal advice and consultation

The best part of writing a book is not—surprise—sitting down at the computer every day in the same old sweats (actually, I alternate). The best part for me is personal interaction with readers like you. I love hearing about your fashion experiences, sharing ideas and insights, and helping you out of a fashion dilemma when I can.

So I've set up two great ways for us to communicate. The first is my website—www.LeahFeldon.com—which is packed with useful information, including regular trend reports, style tips, and good deals when I find them. You can ask me questions via e-mail and get the lowdown on my other books, including the last one, *Dress Like a Million (on Considerably Less)*, which shows how to pull together a great wardrobe without breaking the bank—a great companion book to this one.

For more personalized advice, you can reach me through my **consultation hotline.** Call 615-292-9490 to arrange a time to discuss your individual wardrobe or whatever style concerns or questions you may have. I also keep time in my schedule for a small number of private at-home consultations every year. (Fee schedules are available on request.)

Either way, let's stay in touch. I'd love to hear from you.

Best always,

Leah

LEAH FELDON has been helping women realize their personal best for more than twenty years via her books, television shows, magazine articles, and personal consultations. A former *PM Magazine* cohost and *Today* show contributor, Ms. Feldon has hosted her own series, *Simply Style,* for the Learning Channel and has appeared as a guest commentator on innumerable shows, including the *Oprah Winfrey Show, Extra, Entertainment Tonight,* and *Hard Copy.* She was also a long-time special correspondent for *People* magazine and has served as national media spokesperson for some of America's most notable companies.